LEADING PEER SUPPORT AND SELF-HELP GROUPS: A POCKET RESOURCE FOR PEER SPECIALISTS AND SUPPORT GROUP FACILITATORS

LEADING PEER SUPPORT AND SELF-HELP GROUPS: A POCKET RESOURCE FOR PEER SPECIALISTS AND SUPPORT GROUP FACILITATORS

Charles Drebing, PhD

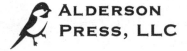

ALDERSON PRESS, LLC

Copyright © 2016 Charles Drebing, PhD
Cover art © 2016 Laurel Holland

All rights reserved.
No part of this book may be photocopied or otherwise
reproduced without written permission.

For information about permission to reproduce selections from
this book, write to:

Alderson Press, LLC
15 Church Place
Holliston, MA 01746

Library of Congress Cataloging in Publication Data
Drebing, Charles, 1959–
Leading Peer Support and Self-Help Groups: A Pocket Resource
for Peer Specialists and Support Group Facilitators/ by
Charles E. Drebing
ISBN 978-1-329-95692-6

This book is dedicated to all of the people who share openly in peer support and self-help groups, providing others with a chance to hear honest words spoken from the heart. Their willingness to tell their personal truths to others, and to listen to and support others struggling to face themselves, makes these groups the invaluable resources they are.

PREFACE

If you are reading this book, you are likely interested in leading—or already do lead—a peer support group. You are one of the hundreds of thousands of individuals worldwide who have stepped up to serve your neighbors by providing the support that self-help groups need. Without your willingness and work, a lot of good would not occur.

This book results from my own work as a manager and researcher in mental health services. As I work at improving these services, I recognize two key factors that point to the need for this book.

First, a large and growing body of research shows that, in addition to all of the common forms of treatment we associate with modern healthcare (drugs, procedures, technology), social support plays a huge role in who recovers from illnesses, who uses healthcare effectively, who enjoys good health (both mentally and physically), and even how long people live. "Social support" is a term that refers to the caring and potential caring we feel from those around us, and it is much more influential in our lives than we usually recognize. For example, the psychologist Julianne Holt-Lunstad and her colleagues (2010) reviewed all of the research studies of the most common predictors of longevity and found that social support is a very powerful predictor—more powerful than obesity, exercise, alcohol consumption, and even tobacco use. Health behaviors like tobacco use and diet get a lot attention in the press, but the more influential factors of social support and community connectedness are usually overlooked.

Secondly, a separate large and growing body of research indicates that the naturally occurring social support we enjoy in our family and community life in the United States has been steadily declining over the past fifty years, both in quantity and quality. In his landmark 2000 book, *Bowling Alone*, political scientist Robert Putnam documents this steady decline in many of the ways that we connect with each other—in community activities, in volunteerism, in time spent together, charitable giving, involvement in community service, in religious organizations. We are less likely to interact with our neighbors, less likely to see them as good people, and less likely to trust them. So the social support that is so important to our individual and community wellness is in much shorter supply than it used to be.

Given these discouraging findings, it was very reassuring when I started looking at the research on peer support and self-help groups. Over the same period of time that community connection across the United States has been declining, the number of people who are attending some form of peer support groups has been growing dramatically. There are now more visits each year to peer support groups than there are to mental health professionals and the numbers are continuing to grow. This is even more surprising (and encouraging) when we remember that there is no profit margin driving this growth—no one makes money off of peer support groups; no one is actively marketing them. The factors that have driven their expansion include the desire people have to connect with others and the benefits they experience from attending support groups as they try to resolve challenging life situations.

So now we have this large movement of peer support that has grown naturally alongside our healthcare system, and as part of our community life. Those who have made this happen are almost all volunteers. They do the work with little fanfare and little professional training or supervision. And the resources to support those taking the lead are very limited. Most materials I have been able to find include just enough information to help someone start a new peer support group and to deal with the most common headaches. Those of us who are mental health professionals know a great deal about how to develop and lead successful groups, but this knowledge has not been translated into useful tools for the hundreds of thousands of people who lead peer support groups each week.

At a personal level, I have also attended a number of peer support groups. I have been deeply impressed by the powerful sense of connectedness and commitment I have seen among the members. In a society that is increasingly thin on opportunities to connect, peer groups can provide people with the experience of a deep sense of community, including opportunities to know others and to be known, to care about others and to be cared about.

As a mental health researcher and administrator, I know that our healthcare system is big, expensive, and riddled with gaps in exactly the areas that peer support groups fill. My hope is to see the number and type of peer support groups continue to grow, and yet I know that for that to happen, we need to find ways to better support those people willing to facilitate those groups. This book is one step toward making that happen.

As someone willing to serve others and the community by leading peer support/self-help groups, you deserve our thanks and our support. We need to provide you with the best information and guidance possible to ensure you can do this important job as well as possible. I know that there are many benefits inherent in the work that you do. My hope is that this book will provide you with some needed tools to make your job easier. I also hope it can make it more likely you can help your group get to the point where you see that you have helped create real community and real connection between your members.

I wish you the best of luck in your important work and welcome feedback about any other information or resources that should be included in a revised version of this book.

Charles Drebing, PhD
March, 2016
CEDrebing@gmail.com

CONTENTS

ACKNOWLEDGMENTS

Special thanks to a host of veterans at the Bedford VA Medical Center who have shown me how peer support groups can be critical for many people's recovery. Tony Russo, Chuck Carroll, and Stuart E. Krentcil are just a few of those whose work with peer support groups has been a source of inspiration for this book. Additional thanks to Laurel Holland for her creative support, Elizabeth Kingfield and Anja Bircher for their help with research, and Heather Rodino for her exceptional input and editorial assistance.

HOW TO USE THIS BOOK

This book is designed to be an easy-to-access resource that you can use while facilitating peer support/self-help groups. It is specifically designed for Peer Specialists and other volunteer leaders/facilitators who manage the wide range of peer support and self-help groups common today, including those focusing on mental health and substance-use issues, medical issues, disabilities, challenging life situations, and any other reason people find to gather to support each other.

Because peer support groups can be challenging to lead, and because those willing to lead them often have relatively limited formal training, this pocket resource is designed to provide some of the basic information about common strategies you need to know in order to be effective. It also includes information and guidance for those who want to develop their skills further and pursue the education and personal development that can help one be a more effective group facilitator.

The book includes a section of specific resource and referral information that support group leaders frequently need to share with the people they support. Some of this information will need to be customized for the setting and locale in which you are working or volunteering. For this reason, you'll be asked to fill in key phone numbers, contacts, referral sources, and other information so that it will be easily available to you while you are working (see Chapter 15).

Appendix A contains a brief summary of recent research findings about the impact of peer support groups. This information has been included both for your own interest and for you to share with potential partners and referral sources that need to better understand the effectiveness of peer support groups in order to be more enthusiastic supporters of them. Finally, appendix B provides a quick guide to dealing with critical situations that you may stumble upon in your work. You will want to keep that section readily available as a reference for those rare but important situations.

This book is not meant to replace information you will need to lead support groups affiliated with specific organizations, and it is not a substitute for learning the guidelines and policies of the organization you work for. It does include additional links and contacts that can help you continue your growth in this important role.

CHAPTER 1

WHAT IS A PEER SUPPORT GROUP AND WHY IS IT VALUABLE?

A <u>Peer Support Group</u>, also described as a "self-help group" or a "mutual aid" or "mutual help" group, refers to a group of people who gather together to talk about shared problems or experiences and to provide informal support to each other. (I will use the terms "peer support group" and "self-help group" interchangeably.) The focus of the group may be a common clinical condition (such as addiction, diabetes, or depression), a life problem (a trauma, loss of child, or bankruptcy), or a personal circumstance or challenge (veterans groups, those trying to lose weight, or people looking to advance their career). The support usually comes in the form of emotional support, information, or guidance based on personal experience. Some groups may have additional agendas, such as advocacy or community service, but all have mutual support as a central activity. While some "support groups" may have a professional facilitator, peer support groups focus on support from non-professional volunteer members.

Peer support groups can take many forms. For example, some meet in-person, while others use a conference call– or web-based format. Some groups are open to drop-in attendance, indicating that anyone who is seeking peer support can attend any meeting; others may be closed, with attendance limited to a specific set of people who are identified as members. While most peer support groups are fairly small in size, allowing everyone a chance to talk, some are quite large or have no size limits. Meeting format can also vary: some groups have a fairly set routine, and others have more unstructured meetings. Participation in some groups is typically just a few meetings in length, while others have members who have been attending for years.

Taken together, peer support groups represent a surprisingly large and growing resource for our communities. <u>More visits are made to peer support groups each year than to all types of mental health professionals combined</u>. Ten to twenty percent of the U.S. population has participated in a peer support group at some time in their lives, with between 5 and 10 percent having participated in the past year. This popularity cannot be attributed to marketing, as these groups generally have little publicity of any kind. Instead, it's due to the tangible benefits that participants receive, the groups' ease of access, and the lack of any formal cost.

Participation in peer support groups has grown dramatically over the past fifty years, both in terms of the number of groups and the scope of issues that these groups deal with. While the largest number of groups continues to be focused around helping participants overcome substance-use problems, growing numbers are organized around very diverse needs and themes. You can now find support groups for almost every medical or mental health issue, most difficult life situations or experiences, and even broad issues of living (such as retirement and career development). Clearly, this is a major development in how we function as a community and how we get and give support in the modern world. It is worth considering some of the specific benefits that participants and researchers have identified.

COMMON BENEFITS

1. <u>Feeling Less Isolated</u>: Feeling isolated or "different" is common when dealing with a clinical or life problem. Gathering with others who are facing the same challenge is a very concrete way to decrease that sense of isolation. Participants in peer support groups often comment about not feeling "so alone" or feeling that they are with people who "understand" them because of the shared experience. In many situations, feeling less alone is the most important step in making a challenge more manageable.

2. <u>Receiving Practical Information Based on Personal Experience</u>: While there are many sources of information to help people deal with almost any life challenge (books, websites, professionals), the information that can be provided by others who have experienced that particular challenge has some unique advantages. It is often more practical and realistic, as it comes from someone who has actually struggled with the problem. It is also easier to have confidence in it, because the individual providing the information usually does not have any financial incentive that might influence what he or she shares.

3. <u>Receiving Emotional Support</u>: We are social animals, and social support is more important to our physical and emotional health than we typically appreciate. Peer support groups are an ideal setting in which people can gather with the explicit purpose of providing and receiving encouragement and affirmation. Most people who attend peer support groups have family and friends who could provide support; however, in many situations and for various reasons, these individuals would rather look outside their

current network for some types of issues and problems. This
may be due to the desire for privacy or because it's sometimes
easier to lean on other people who have the same problem.
Others may find that talking about some topics is more easily
done with "strangers" than with family or friends. Regardless of
the reason, those who attend self-help groups generally find them
to be a special opportunity to receive support from others who
understand what they're going through.

4. <u>Receiving Practical Support</u>: While receiving emotional
support is central to most peer support groups, we should not
overlook the benefits of practical support. As peer support group
relationships develop over time, many members aid each other in
practical ways outside of the meetings. This support can take
many forms, such as giving someone a ride to an appointment,
but it is often just part of what makes group membership
valuable for all.

5. <u>Gaining Insight into How to Deal with a Common Problem</u>:
In most peer support group meetings, attendees talk about how
they are trying to cope with a common challenge they are facing,
and they listen to other attendees do the same. Members often
comment that these discussions give them better insight into
their own challenge, as well as improved strategies for coping
with that challenge.

6. <u>Gaining Broader Insight into Yourself and Your Life</u>:
"Attending a peer support group is like holding a mirror in front
of me—I see myself more clearly by listening to others in the
same situation." This comment by a peer support group member
points to a key benefit for many attendees. We often don't see
ourselves clearly, and peer support groups help us understand
our own experiences and reactions to those experiences. Many
peer support group members also report that being part of a
group helps them see the meaning of those experiences and their

life in a different way. As members talk about the problems they are seeking to overcome, they start to think differently about what the problem means in their lives. This evolving understanding becomes part of the personal growth that many members report as an outcome of being in a group.

7. <u>Gaining a Greater Sense of Control over the Problem</u>: Improved insight and coping strategies usually result in members having a better sense of control in the face of the shared challenge. Such a sense of control is usually associated with lower levels of stress, anxiety, and depression, and high rates of active coping and problem-solving.

8. <u>Expanding or Changing Some of Your Social Network</u>: For those who become regular attendees of a peer support group, the group often becomes part of their network of friends, expanding the number of people they feel supported by. For some peer support groups, like Alcoholics Anonymous (AA), new members are often seeking to replace some of their social network, as they avoid friends and/or family who are associated with the problem they are trying to deal with (drinking, drug use, gambling, etc.). The peer support group provides a way of replacing those connections with new people with the same goal.

9. <u>Using Your Experience to Help Others</u>: Peer support groups involve give-and-take and most members come to value the experience of giving support to others as much as, or sometimes even more than, the experience of receiving it. Many find it particularly satisfying to use their difficult experiences to help others, turning a past problem into something of value.

10. <u>Building/Rebuilding Trust in Others</u>: Peer support groups can be a place where members learn that there are other people out there who are supportive and trustworthy. For some, that is a new lesson—or an important lesson to relearn. Some have few

opportunities to develop relationships with others whom they can trust, and the chance to do so can be a life-changing experience.

PEER SUPPORT GROUPS VS. PSYCHOTHERAPY GROUPS

One of the other common types of groups that people may experience or know about is group psychotherapy. It's worth reviewing some important distinctions between peer support groups and group therapy.

Peer Support Groups	Psychotherapy Groups
Are composed entirely (or almost entirely) of people who have a common life experience or problem. All attendees participate due to their status as peers who share this problem or challenge.	Include one or more licensed clinicians who create and manage a formal clinical experience for a group of people who are "patients" to the provider(s).
May or may not have an identified facilitator. Most facilitators or leaders are not professional clinicians. There is usually not a significant difference between the status and role of the facilitator and the other members.	Are always led by one or more licensed professional clinicians. There is significant difference between the providers and the attendees in terms of status and role.
Because leadership is informal, the facilitators have very limited liability for what happens at the meeting.	Because leaders are licensed professionals, they are responsible for leading the group according to community-based professional standards, and they are liable for their actions.

Peer Support Groups	Psychotherapy Groups
Attendance is voluntary.	While attendance is voluntary, there may also be financial or clinical expectations between the leader and the attendees.
There is usually no cost to attend peer support groups, or any cost is voluntary.	There is usually a cost paid by the attendees and/or their health insurance.
The main benefits come from discussion between peers attending the meeting.	The main benefits come from either discussion between patients attending the meeting or comments and guidance provided by the professional leader.

CHAPTER 2

WHAT DOES A HEALTHY PEER SUPPORT GROUP LOOK LIKE?

Peer support groups can be very diverse, differing in the focus of interest, the size of the group, the format for meetings, and the amount of time spent together. Signs that a group is functioning well can also vary between groups, particularly as a group evolves from a new group into a mature group.

Still, when a peer support group is functioning well, some common markers shine through. Effective leaders learn to recognize and track these signs so that they know when the group may be struggling and need more support, and when a group is doing well and they can relax and let it flourish. The following are some of the signs of a well-functioning peer support group.

COMMUNICATION
The most visible evidence of a healthy peer support group is good communication between members. For example, members typically talk with each other before, during, and after meetings, as well as outside of meetings. In new groups, communication may be slow at the start. The amount of talking may vary

between groups, just like between people, but all healthy peer support groups will be marked by ongoing communication that is valued by the members.

CONNECTION

Healthy groups are marked by more than just communication. People gather so they can connect with each other. Connection can look different in different settings, but here are a few indicators:

- Members communicate about shared interests and experiences beyond the central theme of the group.

- Members show evidence that they are actively listening to each other.

- Members make comments that suggest that they have an impact on each other.

- Members are happy to see each other and happy in each other's presence. Sometimes this is expressed in words, but more commonly you'll see it in the faces and tone of voice of people arriving and leaving meetings.

TRUST AND ACCEPTANCE

Connection is related to how much members feel they can trust each other and the group, and how much they feel they are accepted as individuals in the group. Over time, group members find out both how they are similar to other people in the group—and also how they are different. A healthy group not only supports this discovery but provides a clear message that both the similarities and the differences are good things that enrich the group. The result is that members feel valued as people and not just for how alike they are to everyone else. This feeling of acceptance is one of the most powerful elements of being part of a peer support group, and one that can be most life-changing. This group trait is most evident when members act in a way that shows they trust that other members accept them as individuals, as reflected in the following actions:

- Members share their unique experiences and personal differences.

- Members recognize and appreciate the common and unique experiences of others.

- Members take risks in what they share and do. Because they trust that other members accept and care about them, they are willing to be increasingly open in what they share and willing to act in new ways in the group.

WANTING TO BE TOGETHER

A healthy group almost always becomes a valuable experience for the members, and so they want to come to meetings and be with the other group members. You will observe that:

- People are attached to the group. They put out effort and make sacrifices to come to the meetings. They make comments about looking forward to coming and express disappointment when they cannot.

- Members are attached to other members. They put out effort and make sacrifices to talk and spend time with each other outside of the meeting.

- Members feel that they make a significant contribution to the group and that their participation matters.

SELF-DISCLOSURE

Any support group leader should track the degree to which members talk openly about their personal experiences. Groups with low levels of trust tend to talk about emotionally safe topics, such as information and facts, providers and healthcare systems, and issues external to the group. When trust levels are high, however, they'll talk about their own lives, their struggles and successes, and parts of their experience that they may not fully understand. They may also talk about what is going on in the group, including their feelings about and conflicts with other members, if they feel hurt or supported, and so on. In a healthy group, other members respond to this type of self-disclosure with recognition, support, and further self-disclosure.

GIVING AND RECEIVING SUPPORT

In a well-functioning peer support group, most members will be involved in both receiving and giving support. This support may take the form of sharing information or strategies, relating experiences, or expressing care and concern. While some members will naturally have more to give or be naturally more generous, and others will have times of greater need, everyone needs to get involved in both giving and receiving. When many members only give—or only receive—support, the group is not functioning well. Peer support needs to be mutual.

MOVEMENT AND EXPLORATION

Because members feel trust in a healthy functioning group, their growing self-disclosure and willingness to take risks create movement in what the group talks about and deals with. Often, leaders will see a steady deepening of what members will be willing to share. The topics of discussion may change in content and theme, as members explore new areas of concern together. If there is a good level of trust, members will be more willing to talk about topics they don't fully understand and those that feel confusing or threatening. These discussions often break new ground, as the group explores new areas of experience.

CONNECTIONS BETWEEN MEMBERS AND THE LEADER

Connections between individual group members and between individual members and the whole group are key to the value of peer support groups. While group leaders play an important role, and hold a particularly important place in some members' feelings about the group, their role is not - or at least should not- be more important than the role of other group members. When a group is starting, or when new members are joining, the group leader can be the person whom most people know and feel attached to. And at key times, the leader may play a particularly important part in helping a group deal with a challenge, and so may be seen by members as particularly valuable. If, however, this person is always the primary focus of connection with the group, then the group has not developed into a well-functioning peer support group. This can be a sign that the group has not provided enough caring and support to its members. It may also indicate that the leader has not done enough to help the members support each other, but has instead stayed too long in the center of the group.

CHAPTER 3

UNDERSTANDING YOUR ROLE: WHAT "LEADERSHIP" MEANS IN A PEER SUPPORT GROUP

The term "leadership" can mean many different things depending on the situation. The Merriam-Webster dictionary defines the term "leader" as one who "guides" or "conducts." There are many ways of guiding or conducting a group of people. In settings like a hospital emergency room, effective leadership means exerting a high degree of control over what others do and providing strong direction so that a team can respond quickly and effectively to meet their goal of successfully handling emergencies. In other settings, the group's goal is different and so leadership has to be different. For example, if a peer support group leader were as active and controlling as the leader of an emergency room team, no one would want to come to a meeting, and little growth would occur. In this instance, effective leadership means that you function in a way that facilitates the functioning of a healthy peer support group, as described in the last chapter. To do so, effective leaders "guide" and "conduct" the group in a way that achieves the following:

CREATING A SUPPORTIVE ENVIRONMENT

An effective leader helps create an environment in which successful peer support grows. Such an environment includes the following:

- <u>A Predictable Setting</u>: Try to ensure that (a) meetings start on time, (b) the physical location is consistently clean and comfortable, (c) the focus of the meeting is consistent, and (d) the format is consistent.

- <u>A Safe Setting</u>: There can be potential dangers in peer support groups, and so effective leaders work to ensure that the group is safe for people to participate in. To do so, leaders ensure that members are not allowed, for example, to treat each other poorly or be disrespectful. Leaders are particularly careful when strong emotions arise, and may step in to ensure they are managed safely. When the group stumbles, effective leaders ensure that it is recognized and corrective action is taken, including any needed repair work. Leaders keep an eye out for members and potential members who may have such significant psychiatric and/or personality issues that they pose a risk to the safety of the group. While this is rare, it does occur, and leaders are responsible for taking action (see chapter 4 for more guidance on those situations).

- <u>A Caring Setting</u>: Set the tone so that everyone understands that in the group, people are valued and that connection is very important. While groups may work on tasks together, such as studying a book or developing a service project, the task is never so important that the mutual support between members becomes secondary. This caring and respect should be consistent and be for everyone—not just those who are most popular, most active, have been in the group the longest, or most respected.

EMPHASIZING THE PARTICIPATION OF GROUP MEMBERS: GIVING THE MESSAGE THAT WHAT OTHERS SAY IS MORE IMPORTANT THAN WHAT THE LEADER SAYS

New peer group facilitators sometimes make the mistake of thinking that what they say in the group is more important than what others say. People rarely say that they benefit from peer support groups primarily because of the insights that the leader shared. It is much more likely that they will benefit from the relationships with others, and the chance to share and to listen to others. When leaders talk too much or talk in a way that emphasizes their role or wisdom, they compete with the focus on the members. Experienced leaders know that in many situations, they will be most effective by being quiet or by encouraging others to talk. Even when the leader may have wonderful insights to share, he or she knows that it is more important for others to talk in order for the group to move forward.

MODELING GOOD PARTICIPATION

One of the most important roles peer group leaders have is as a model of how a good member acts. Their behavior provides guidance for those members who don't have much experience in healthy peer support groups, and helps push the group toward sharing more openly. To be a good model, leaders should:

- Arrive at meetings on time, stay until the end, and follow the group's guidelines
- Share openly about their experiences
- Listen actively to others and interact with their comments
- Express support and respect for others
- Take risks in sharing more openly as the group becomes more trustworthy in how they respond.

ENCOURAGING BUT NOT FORCING CONNECTION

Attendance in peer support groups is almost always voluntary. People are attracted to them because they want to be part of a group—to share their experiences and connect with others. How much they share depends mostly on the degree of trust the group builds: the greater the trust, the greater the sharing and connection.

Leaders who push members to make connections or to share openly often have the opposite effect: people become defensive and less likely to share. Pushy leaders also often reduce the sense of trust the group feels. Inviting and encouraging sharing and connection is very different from forcing it. It is never appropriate to force people to share about something they do not want to talk about.

RECOGNIZING THAT THE GROUP IS RESPONSIBLE

New peer group leaders often make the mistake of feeling and acting as though they hold primary responsibility for how the group develops. If the group doesn't go well, they feel they have failed. And if it does, they feel responsible for its success. While the leader has a special role, it is important to recognize that it is the group that is responsible for what happens: the members make decisions about what they will say or do. To the degree that the leader communicates this responsibility to them, members will take it on. Leaders who directly or indirectly communicate that they feel responsible for the success of the group will encourage members not to feel responsible and so not act in a responsible way.

Ways leaders can communicate that the group is responsible for its own development include:

- Asking the group to set up the basic framework of how to work together, including initial guidelines about expectations, activities, etc.: "What will be the basic guidelines for our meetings?"
- Asking the group to make most decisions that come up: "What does the group want to do about meeting over the holidays?"
- Commenting on the group's actions in a way that communicates their responsibility: "The group seems undecided about what we talk about tonight. What do we want to do about that?"
- Avoid comments that emphasize the leader's role, such as "When I started this group..." or "As the leader, I know that we should..."

LEADERSHIP AS A SHARED ACTIVITY

Leadership in a peer support group should be shared—and not be the function of one person alone. For the health of the group you want as many people as possible to feel some sense of responsibility for how the group is going and to feel able and willing to contribute to its leadership. You primarily accomplish this by communicating this expectation, both directly and indirectly, to the group. For example, ask members to take on leadership tasks. When the members don't act as though they hold some responsibility for supporting and organizing the group, ask them why not. Help them to see that the entire group is needed to make this happen.

A second element that ensures that leadership is shared is your effort to develop and support a co-leader. All groups should have at least two identified leaders if at all possible. Co-leaders provide a number of practical benefits: They back each other up in case of illness. They offer different perspectives on challenging situations facing the group. They share some of the work that can drain a single leader. And, they offer different leadership strengths to the group.

LEADERSHIP AS SERVICE

An emerging model of leadership is the idea of "leader as servant," a model that is now popular in business leadership and fits very well with peer support group leadership. The term "Servant as Leader" was coined by Robert Greenleaf, a businessman-turned-writer, in an essay in 1970. He points out that while many people seek leadership roles out of a desire to exercise power or influence, the primary concern of a servant leader is the welfare of those they serve. Greenleaf writes: "The difference manifests itself in the care taken by the servant—first to make sure that other people's highest priority needs are being served. The best test, and difficult to administer, is: Do those served grow as persons? Do they, while being served, become healthier, wiser, freer, more autonomous, more likely themselves to become servants?"

This model of leadership is central to healthy peer support group leadership. Directive leadership (telling others what to do, trying to control what happens) does not work with peer support groups and will often cripple or destroy a healthy support group. The leader must focus on serving the group and acting in a way that promotes the members' involvement in the group process.

COMMON MISTAKES TO AVOID

It is worthwhile considering a few of the most common mistakes that peer support group leaders fall into.

1. Feeling Too Responsible for How the Group Goes. As noted earlier, an effective leader believes and acts as though the group is responsible for the meeting and for what happens in the group. When leaders start to act or feel that they are responsible, a

number of common problems begin to show up: The group members start acting as though the leader is responsible— and so they don't take responsibility. They tend to work less, to engage less, and to enjoy the group less. There is less vitality in the group and usually more frustration with the leader, who is felt to hold all of the control and the "answers."

2. <u>Speaking Too Much</u>. A mistake related to feeling too responsible is talking too much. Members benefit most from the opportunities they have to engage in genuine discussion with other members. Leaders who speak more than other members in the meeting often are trying too hard to control the meeting or taking too much responsibility for how the meeting goes.

3. <u>Pushing Too Hard</u>. In general, group members will create connections as they feel more comfortable and trusting of others. When members are pushed to do this, they naturally react by resisting such connections. You cannot rush the process of learning to trust others, and if you try to force it, the impact is likely to be negative. Effective peer support group leaders help create an environment and then let the natural processes of connection and trust-building occur.

4. <u>Acting Like a Therapist</u>. Peer support groups are not therapy groups and much of the wonderful work that occurs there is different from what occurs in therapy groups. A leader who acts like a therapist is undermining the group. Examples of this include leaders who act like they are not members of the group, leaders who frequently make clinical interpretations of members' comments, leaders who frequently refer to their own clinical knowledge as an authority, and leaders who present themselves as aligned with, or extensions of, clinical providers.

5. <u>Doing Too Much Behind the Scenes</u>. In most groups a range of practical things needs to be done to make sure everything runs smoothly: coffee needs to be made, chairs need to be set up, members need to be called, and conversations need to be followed up on. Some leaders fall into the trap of feeling that if they don't do these tasks, no one will. In fact, the opposite is true—if *they* do them, *then* no one else will. Part of the benefit of the group is getting drawn into contributing to it in some way. While members are often initially ambivalent about contributing, a part of them wants and needs to do so if they are to feel truly connected to the group.

A FINAL NOTE ON BEING A LEADER

Being a peer support group leader is primarily a way to serve others by helping to create a safe, comfortable setting for members to connect with other people and to give and receive support. Service to others as a leader is rewarding, but can also take a lot of time and energy outside of the meeting itself, including that range of tasks needed to manage the meetings, ensuring that new members are being recruited, saying goodbye to departing members, and coordinating practical elements such as refreshments and meeting space. Support group leadership also takes a lot of internal work as well, as you reflect on how the group is doing, what it needs, how the meetings are affecting you emotionally, and what your psychological needs are with respect to the group.

Being a group leader has some wonderful benefits. Leaders always learn a lot about themselves and other people. Groups are a wonderful place to learn about the human psyche and experience. Group leaders learn valuable facilitation and support skills that can be applied to many other situations at work or in their personal life. They also get to meet a lot of wonderful people, and have a chance to give and receive support.

Overall, peer support group leaders have the satisfaction of knowing that they have helped create opportunities for people to be open and honest with each other and to build connections in an increasingly disconnected world. Social scientists have been documenting the many ways in which opportunities for human connection are steadily declining in modern Western culture (Putnam, 2000). The increasing use of peer support groups may be a partial answer that that troubling trend. By serving as a peer support group leader, you are helping to create those opportunities that our communities need.

CHAPTER 4

KEY SKILLS FOR FACILITATING A GROUP MEETING

Group meetings can vary widely depending on the type of peer support group. For example, 12-step meetings look fairly different from support groups for expectant mothers. Regardless of the format and focus, a leader needs a number of key skills to help develop and support a successful meeting.

SETTING UP THE MEETING

Leaders often start a peer support group meeting in some way that either reflects the shared rituals of the group (e.g., AA has specific practices for the opening of meetings) or the goal and practices that the individual group has decided upon. As the leader, you want to be aware of any such established practices or expectations and follow that routine. Groups often like to start with these routines or rituals because they are ways of reminding everyone, including new members, what the meeting is about and what to expect. It is a concrete way to indicate that the meeting has started and that members need to shift their attention and behavior to the work at hand.

<u>Goals and Comfort Agreements</u>: It is common for many groups to start each meeting with a review of the basic goal for the meeting and the guidelines (sometimes referred to as a "Comfort Agreement") they have set for how they will act. The guidelines help everyone to remember what the meeting is about, what is expected of them, and how the group will work together to ensure that the meeting is safe and productive. While groups create a wide variety of guidelines, there are some common elements in many comfort agreements:

- Be respectful to everyone
- No personal attacks
- Disagreements are OK but respect the person
- Avoid interpreting others' feelings
- Speak for yourself
- No cross-talking, no sidebar conversations
- Try not to interrupt; try not to talk so long that others will feel a need to interrupt you
- Meetings will start and end on time
- Respect physical boundaries—don't hug or touch without asking permission first
- Try to avoid talking about your religious or political views in a way that may make others uncomfortable; no proselytizing
- Everyone's cellphones should be silenced
- If attendees need to leave early, they should do so without disrupting the meeting

A comment about confidentiality is also common, usually something to the effect of "What is shared in this group stays in this group." You will want to ask group members for their commitment to confidentiality and then include that specific agreement in the group's comfort agreement.

Some additional issues you may want to ask the group about include:

- Whether members are allowed to take photographs of meetings.
- Who is able to attend a meeting. Some groups allow family members and friends, while others limit attendance to only people who meet certain criteria.
- How members should communicate with the group leader(s) outside of the meeting.
- If there will be any funds used for anything and how those funds will be collected and managed.

Personal Introductions: Some groups start by having all attendees introduce themselves, giving their name and sharing something about themselves, either related to the purpose of the group (e.g., "Tell us the reason you came to the meeting") or something that might start conversation or connections (e.g., "Say something unique about yourself" or "Say something about you that no one in the room knows"). In large groups, personal introductions can take a large amount of time and so may need to be very brief or even omitted entirely.

Personal Check-Ins: Some groups start meetings by having members "check-in" by giving the group an update on how they are doing with respect to the reason for the meeting, such as "How are you doing with your job search?" or "What has been happening with your efforts to reduce your gambling?" This ritual quickly gets the meeting focused on the work of the group and encourages everyone to talk early. However, leaders may need to help ensure individual check-ins do not go too long.

Reading Key Content: Some groups start with a reading that helps focus the group on their work and/or the topic of discussion for that particular meeting. As group leader, you may be expected to select the reading and to read it to the group. This is often a good task to share with other group members to encourage them to be more involved. Readings can be dictated by the organization, but when you have discretion, ensure that the reading is clear, focused, and long enough to introduce the topic but not so long or complex that it detracts from the discussion.

Stating Common Shared Beliefs: Similar to reading key content, some groups start by reading a shared set of beliefs or goals. Again, sometimes this reading is dictated by the larger organization, but other times the group has some discretion. This method has the advantage of focusing attention on how the group members are to do the work of the group. It can also give a sense of shared vision, and build hope that these beliefs will lead to success.

Setting and/or Reviewing Agendas: A meeting can also start by setting a specific agenda or reviewing an agenda set previously by the group or the leader. Again, this opening ritual helps the group focus quickly on what they have to do in their meeting, and builds hope by setting goals and providing structure for the meeting.

MANAGING THE DISCUSSION DURING THE MEETING: BASIC SKILLS

The main part of the meeting typically involves either focused or open discussion by group members. While members will do most of the talking, the leader has the important role of helping the discussion stay on track and making sure members follow the agreed-upon tenets of the group's comfort agreement. This is often not an easy task, and takes a number of skills that leaders develop over time. They include some of the following:

<u>Modeling Good Participation</u>: Good leaders model what it means to be a good group member. They come on time and leave on time. They follow the comfort agreement. They contribute comments that reflect their membership in the group. They listen well to others, trying to hear what the other person is really saying. They respond with support, humor, and honesty in a way that is helpful and authentic.

<u>Self Disclosure by the Leader: Contributing, but Not Too Much</u>: As members, leaders should contribute to the discussion as much as other members, including comments about their own personal experiences and views. The tone of the comments should also be similar to that of other members. Be sure to avoid comments that draw attention to your role as a leader and sound different from those of other members.

<u>Keeping the Discussion Focused</u>: All group meetings have the potential to lose focus. Members may want to talk about unrelated topics, or they may make long and rambling comments that leave the group feeling bored or frustrated. Effective leaders find ways to gently nudge the group back on track with simple comments that bend the discussion back to the group's mission, or by helping draw others into a response to a long or confusing comment. It is important to act before the discussion has gotten so far off-track that there is a great deal of frustration in the room. It is also important to do so in a way that is respectful to the member(s) who has lost focus. Often something like:

- "I can see that this is important for you, John, and I wonder how this fits with . . ."
- "Bill, I wonder if you have thoughts about this topic."

When a member or members are more insistent on talking about topics unrelated to the group's mission, the leader may need to take more obvious steps, including:

- Drawing the group's attention to the fact that the discussion has gotten away from the agenda and asking the group to discuss this.
- Talking with the individual(s) outside of the group about the need to stay on topic.

Identifying Common Themes: Members often share common experiences, which are reflected in comments they make during meetings. It is often helpful for members to recognize those commonalities, as it helps to further break their sense of isolation and often spurs more discussion about shared experiences. Effective leaders are quick to recognize those commonalities and to point them out when such a comment will move the discussion forward.

Balancing the Needs of the Individual Group Member with the Needs of the Group As a Whole: In one sense, when people form a group, that group becomes an entity that has an identity and dynamics of its own. As such, groups have needs that may be different from some of the needs of the individual members. An effective group leader will keep an eye on the needs and behaviors of the individual attendees as well as those of the group. Examples of group needs include:

- A Group That Needs Focus. This is often shown when members' comments are not focused on the target of the group and drift to other issues.
- A Group That Needs Structure. This is often shown when members break boundaries in little ways (e.g., being late, having sidebar discussions) or in big ways (e.g., breaking confidentiality, being overtly disrespectful).
- A Group That Needs Added Support. This can be seen when members talk about difficult situations in ways that are too risky or that create dangers of significant destructive conflict.

An effective leader not only recognizes the importance of
balancing the needs of individuals with the needs of the group,
but can help members recognize this as well.

Balancing Other Areas of Group Discussion: With experience,
you will notice when the discussion is getting "out of balance" in
one way or another. You and the rest of the group will want to
recognize these situations and help the discussion stay
productive. Here are few things to attend to:

    1. Balancing Which Members Are The Focus of Discussion.
There is a basic assumption in peer support groups that
everyone shares in the giving and receiving of care, including
being the focus of the discussion. Some members will be
more comfortable talking and may tend to dominate
discussion. The group may need help from you in keeping
the right balance, so that less outgoing members have a
chance to speak.

    2. Balancing Between Focusing on a Specific Topic and
Looking at a Variety of Topics. At times you may notice that
the discussion has gotten very focused on a specific topic,
and it may stay on that topic for some time. Be aware that a
limited focus can drain some of the vitality out of a
discussion over time, as other topics are left unexplored. This
problem can be easily addressed with a comment like, "We've
been talking about this for some time. I'm wondering if there
are other topics that we need to focus on as well."

    3. Balancing Between Talking About Painful, Stressful, Sad
Experiences, and Talking About Ways to Cope with Those
Experiences. If the discussion focuses almost exclusively on
the difficult experiences of members, a sense of
discouragement and hopelessness can develop. On the other
hand, when the discussion focuses only on ways of coping

and successful experiences of coping, the discussion will likely be missing a sense of personal connection. When the discussion alternates between both, members have a sense of connection and support in the face of challenging experiences, as well as optimism and interest in ways of successfully dealing with those challenges. You can bring in the topic of coping with a comment like, "I wonder how group members have successfully coped with these experiences in the past." Difficult experiences can be approached by saying something such as, "We've talked a lot about how people cope with the challenges you face, but I wonder if we could hear more about what those challenges feel like for group members."

Like a good meal, a good group discussion will have some balance in the content and type of discussion. Helping keep this balance should not require heavy-handed action, but rather some subtle nudging and suggesting of topics or questions.

Humor is another ingredient that is often found in healthy group discussions, though it varies depending on the group members. In the right amount, however, it can help lighten a discussion and be a way to cope with a challenging topic together.

Talking About What is Happening in the Meeting—what is happening between members—is another occasional element in healthy group talk. This is called "here-and-now talk" because members discuss what is happening in the room at that moment. Sometimes this takes the form of expressing appreciation toward, and caring for other members. Other times, it can be a way of discussing feelings of anger or hurt. Here-and-now talk is valuable in that it feels particularly honest and often more intense than other discussion. The intensity can also make group members more anxious, so be attentive to how they are reacting.

 <u>Knowing When to Be Quiet</u>. Silence is a common part of any conversation and group meeting. People are generally uncomfortable with silence and will often rush to fill it with a comment, often any comment, in order to end it. While groups don't get together to be quiet with each other, the tendency to say anything in order to avoid silence can be a problem. This problem is particularly true for leaders, who often feel that silence is a sign that the meeting is not going well. When leaders make comments simply to fill a quiet moment, it often represents a lost opportunity for the group to take a few moments to think about what they want to say. The experienced leader knows to be patient with silences and let the group sit with them. If silence becomes a large part of the meeting, it may be worth inviting the group to talk about that—how it feels and why it might be happening.

<u>Summarizing</u>. There are times when it is helpful for the group to hear a summary of what they have been talking about. A good summary gives them a sense of the range of topics they have been covering, can tie the topics together in a meaningful way that they don't currently see, and serves as a way to either close discussion on a particular topic or to transition to another topic. Regardless of the reason, leaders are often in a position to make summary comments or to ask other members to try to summarize the discussion. A good summary statement is neither so short that it doesn't really include much of the significant topics, or so long that members have trouble making sense of it.

MANAGING THE DISCUSSION: RESPONDING TO RISKY SITUATIONS

<u>Vulnerable Moments</u>. Experienced leaders know that key moments arise in group meetings that may require a special response by the leader. An effective leader watches for those moments and decides at that time whether or not to respond.

Some common vulnerable moments include: <u>A Member Is in Crisis</u>. During a meeting, it may become clear to the leader, and potentially to the group, that a member is in a personal crisis. This may be as obvious as someone saying he is in a crisis or describing his situation as being chaotic or upsetting. It may also be less obvious. When people are in crisis, they often report feeling overwhelmed by the challenges they face and hopeless about resolving the issue. They may show a lot of emotion—or no emotion at all—but the emotions they do show are usually different than what is typical for that person.

There are several common responses to a member in crisis. What you do as the leader depends on the situation you face:

<u>When There Is Evidence That the Person Is Not Safe</u>. In some crises, people get desperate and some may even be at risk for hurting themselves or others. Appendix A includes common steps that leaders should respond to safety concerns.

- <u>When the Person Is Able to Talk Effectively About How She Is Doing, and the Group Is Able to Respond With Appropriate Support</u>. For many people, the group can provide the support they need while in crisis, and so the leader should simply let the group do its work. If that is not the case, the leader may need to take a more active role.

- <u>When the Person Is Able to Talk Effectively About How He Is Doing but the Group Is Not Able to Respond</u>. It is not uncommon that most or all of the members of a group will not respond, or not respond well, to a member in crisis. You will see evidence of this if no one says anything to the individual, or if the group discussion shifts focus to another topic. Lack of response may be due either to the group not knowing what to do or feeling overwhelmed. In this situation, the leader needs to step in, first to see if she can help the group start to help, or, if it is clear that the group cannot respond, to provide a response.

- <u>When the Person Is Not Able to Talk Effectively About the Crisis</u>. In this situation, the leader may need to become active to help the person to talk about the crisis, or to defer the discussion until later. The leader has a responsibility to keep both individual members and the group as a whole safe, and so he needs to watch for and respond to any issues related to safety. At the same time, the leader wants the group to do as much of the work as possible, and so leaders typically wait to see how the group responds to the crisis before taking on a more active role. If the group responds effectively, that is a good outcome. If they need some encouragement or guidance to respond effectively, that is still a very good outcome. If they are not able to respond, the leader will typically want to step in, either by responding actively in the meeting, or by asking the member in crisis to talk separately either during ("Let's step outside for a moment to talk more about this") or after the meeting ("I wonder if you'd be willing to stay after the meeting so that we can talk more about this individually?").

<u>Someone Is Visibly Upset</u>: A related situation is when someone in the group is not in a crisis, but is still very emotional—very tearful, angry, etc. Emotions, at times intense emotions, come up in peer support groups. In general, this can be a very good thing if the emotions are related to the issues the group is supposed to talk about, and if there is a good response to the individuals expressing the emotions (typically, emotional comments lead to

more discussion). Effective leaders also know that group discussions that include strong emotions can be volatile and even dangerous for the group if the emotion becomes so intense that the group members become afraid or overwhelmed. Thoughtful discussion and expressions of emotion are key in any good peer support group, but they need to be balanced in order to be helpful. If too much emotion is expressed, many group members will feel overwhelmed and will want to stop coming. And if there is a great deal of thoughtful discussion, but very little emotion, many group members may feel the meetings are not actually focusing on things that are important or that they care about, or that there is not enough personal connection. When the discussion can alternate fluidly between the expression of emotion and thoughtful discussion, the balance usually works in a way that helps the group not only to talk about feelings, but also to think them through, such that learning and growth are the result.

Again, the leader's specific response to a member who is quite emotional in a meeting depends on the situation:

- <u>When the Person Is Talking Effectively About the Issue Underlying the Emotion and the Group Is Responding Well by Continuing to Interact with Comments</u>. In this situation the leader should let the group do its work.

- <u>When the Person Is Talking Effectively About Intense Feelings, but the Group Is Having Trouble Responding Effectively</u>. At times, intense emotion will result in a group getting very quiet. Like the member in crisis, the member who is expressing emotion may not get the support or response that is helpful. In this situation, the leader may want to try to encourage the group to respond—to talk about what is being said or felt.

Sometimes it is helpful to simply make the observation about how the group is responding ("Since Mr. Johnson has gotten very upset, the group has gotten very quiet").

- <u>When the Person Is Not Able to Talk Effectively About Feelings, or the Feelings Are About Something That Is Off-Topic</u>. Again, the leader wants the group to deal either with someone having trouble verbalizing feelings or talking off-topic. One strategy is to simply make an observation of this fact and let the group respond. The leader may also step in to help the person clarify her feelings, or to help remind her what the guidelines are for what the group is discussing.

<u>Someone Is Making a Comment That Could Trigger Distress in Other Members</u>. On occasion, a member's comments will include content that could trigger a very bad response from one or more group members. For example, in a group for people who have suffered child abuse, a member may start to describe his experience of child abuse in such detail that other members could begin to re-experience their own traumas. When comments by one member make other members feel so badly that they aren't benefiting from or don't want to come to the group, the leader must address the problem. Often leaders can do this with a simple question like, "I wonder how these comments are affecting other group members," and letting the group explain that the comments are too upsetting. Other times, the leader needs to be more direct, stating something like, "I appreciate how powerful this experience has been for you, but I think these comments are actually too intense for other members right now. Can we step back from this story and talk about. . . ?"

<u>Someone Is Being Attacked</u>. Conflict is a natural part of any peer support group, but it can be destructive, particularly if it leads to

open and aggressive conflict in which one or more members feel that they are being personally attacked, insulted, or disrespected. It is important for groups to know that such comments are against the comfort agreement or group guidelines. Groups and group leaders need to enforce those guidelines, and so should quickly step in to discussions in which members are breaking this rule to stop open conflict and encourage members to talk in a way that is respectful and leads to resolution.

The goal is not to avoid conflict, but to always encourage the group members to either (1) accept that the differences are there and that they can live with those differences or (2) talk about the conflict in a respectful, open manner with the hope that the discussion will lead to better understanding and the reduction or resolution of the conflict. The effective leader is aware of the conflicts present in any given group and is quick to step in to ensure that those that threaten to be destructive are managed in a productive way. The group relies on you to do this, and their trust in the group will grow as they come to know that you will not allow such destructive interactions to occur.

At times, the conflicts are significant enough that the leader will want to ask the key parties to talk outside of the group meeting, either with or without a mediator. This saves the group from spending a large amount of time on the conflict and can give the parties a chance to talk more directly about the issue and hopefully resolve it.

<u>Someone Is Attacking the Group</u>. Less common is the situation in which a member makes comments that openly attack the entire group. This is more than just criticizing the group, which is not necessarily a bad thing; instead, this person makes angry comments that are more focused on damaging the group and/or members than on identifying problems that can be solved. In

these situations, it is again better if the group can respond to the attack in a reasonable and productive way, but this is often not possible. In that case, the effective leader should be fairly quick to respond, and the appropriate response will often start with a request to avoid attacking comments and then asking that the member restate her concerns in more respectful terms ("That type of comment is not really helpful, as you are attacking the group but not saying directly what you are unhappy about and what you would like to see the group do differently"). If the person can do so, the leader can then help the group talk this through. If not, the leader may need to be even more assertive and ask the person to take the conversation outside of the meeting, and to bring it to a special meeting just with the leader. In the long run, if a member is (1) so unhappy with a group that she feels a need to openly attack the group, and (2) unable to resolve the issue with open discussion, then it is typically reasonable for the leader to encourage the member to consider why she would come to a group she is so unhappy with, and to encourage her to look for a new group that better meets her needs.

MANAGING THE DISCUSSION: RESPONDING TO OPPORTUNITIES FOR THE GROUP TO GO DEEPER

Groups, like people, are typically ambivalent about talking honestly about important topics and looking at them at a deeper level. They may in fact wish to do so but feel anxious about what will happen if they do. The effective group leader needs to recognize when opportunities arise for the group to talk more deeply, and when the group is hesitating to do so. At those points, leaders may want to step in to help the group take that next step. Signs that the discussion could go deeper include the following:

<u>Multiple Members Are Talking About the Same Issue</u>. A simple marker of an opportunity to go deeper is when several members are talking about or keep returning to the same issue. Sometimes different members talk about the topic in different ways, or from different perspectives, but they are still working on the same theme. Other times they return to the theme over the course of the same meeting, or even from meeting to meeting. The leader may want to draw the group's attention to this fact with a simple observation and/or added comment, encouraging the group to talk more about the topic.

Some examples of a simple observation would include:
- "Seems like many of us are talking about this topic tonight."
- "These comments sound a lot like our conversation from last week."

Some examples of an added comment to encourage more discussion would include:
- "I'm wondering who else has been having this experience."
- "I wonder if there is more about this issue that we could be saying."

<u>The Discussion Goes Only So Far</u>. A subtler marker that the conversation could go deeper is when the discussion only goes so far, and stops before a logical next step is taken. This situation is tricky to identify, as a discussion can go in many different directions. However, when it shows a pattern over time that suggests that the group is avoiding certain topics or avoiding the next step in the discussion, the leader may want to invite the members to talk about this. Some examples of comments that would invite deeper discussion include:
- "Seems like this is a pattern for our discussions; we talk

about this until we get to this topic, but then don't go any further. Any thoughts about why we might do this?"

- "I wonder if we are avoiding the next step in this conversation. Is there some reason we may not want to talk about the next step?"

Other Dimensions of the Topic Are Not Included in the Discussion, e.g., the Discussion Includes Only the Downside of Something and Not the Benefit, or Only the Benefit and Not the Downside. Sometimes a group may only talk about one side of a topic, such as the benefits of an action but not its risks or costs. If the leader feels that the group may benefit from talking about this other side, a simple observation or invitation is often enough to bring this into the meeting. An example of an invitation would be, "We seem to only talk about the benefits. I'm wondering if anyone has any thoughts about the costs."

CLOSING THE MEETING

Like the rituals and practices that groups use to start a meeting, the ways that groups end their meetings have a number of functions. Often they're a way of signaling that people need to refocus their attention on saying goodbye and getting ready to leave. They may also help members focus on what they will do as a result of the discussion—what actions they will take before the next meeting or as a result of what they learned. They may focus on encouraging hope in members regarding going back to their daily lives. They may also encourage group members to come back next time or to support each other until the next meeting. Some examples of closing rituals include:

Check-Ins. Some groups close meetings by asking members to check-in by telling the group what they are feeling or thinking as they leave the meeting. This gives every member an opportunity to make a last comment. It also gives the leaders an opportunity to see how each person is doing as he or she leaves, and to identify anyone who may be struggling.

Readings. Some groups end with a reading from a key book or source. This brings members back to a common focus and can add an opportunity for reflection.

Stating Common Shared Beliefs. Some groups end by stating shared beliefs, usually by reading a written statement that summarizes how they think about what they are trying to do. This practice can also bring members back to shared beliefs and send them out of the meeting focused on some ideas for the coming week.

Stating "Takeaways" or Goals. Another closing ritual is to end by having members talk about what they learned, will remember from the meeting, or what actions they will take as a result of the meeting. Takeaways can serve as a way to summarize the discussion, to focus the members on applying what they have talked about, and to let the leader know how members experienced the meeting—how helpful it was and what topics were seen as particularly helpful.

Reviewing What Is Coming Up—Next Meetings and Events. Some groups close their meetings by reviewing next steps: when the next meeting is, what events may be happening between now and the next meeting, etc. This ritual is particularly helpful in re-orienting members back to their daily lives, where they also have to focus on their schedule and upcoming events. It also communicates the fact that the group will continue.

FOLLOWING UP WHEN NECESSARY

Group life continues after the meeting, and the effective leader follows up with other members as a way of supporting them. All members should follow up, but the leader often is the model for this behavior. Examples of situations to consider following-up outside the meeting include when:

- Someone leaves the meeting particularly upset
- Someone leaves the meeting clearly ambivalent about attending the group
- Someone mentions that an important event will occur before the next meeting; the event could be particularly difficult or stressful, or it could be particularly good

CHAPTER 5

UNDERSTANDING AND MAINTAINING BOUNDARIES

The concept of boundaries is a very useful tool that will help you and the people you work with avoid confusion and problems within relationships. The basic principle is that we all belong to a number of separate groups, each of which has a separate role and responsibility. "Boundaries" refers to the psychological understanding of those separate roles that we want to maintain, which help us all be clear on what we each are responsible for.

Boundary crossings occur when one or more people act in a way that violates one of the agreed-upon boundaries, or in a way that is "out of bounds." Boundary crossings are not uncommon in life, but often result in confusion and conflict. Difficulty maintaining boundaries has been associated with a number of mental health conditions, and occurs in peer support groups, so you want to be particularly careful to attend to and guard boundaries within any groups you facilitate.

COMMON BOUNDARIES

Boundaries exist in many forms, but the most common include:

The Boundary Between Each Individual: Each person is a separate individual who is responsible for his or her own actions. When we act as though we are responsible for others' actions or they are responsible for ours, problems often ensue.

The Boundary Around a Group of People, Such As an Established Peer Support Group: People who see themselves as a group have a psychological boundary that identifies them as such. This boundary may be subtle and not explicit. Other people may act as though the group is not a group; for example, they may move into the group without even recognizing it. Group members may also act as though the group does not have boundaries; when a member violates group expectations of confidentiality, for example, that person is breaking the group boundary.

The Boundary Between a Person Receiving Formal Healthcare or Social Services and the Provider of Those Services: The boundary between providers and their clients/patients is one of the most important. When clients and providers break these boundaries by becoming romantically involved or socializing outside of treatment, the clinical work typically suffers. Boundary crossings between providers and clients are seen as a serious professional, ethical, and at times, legal breach, and can result in very serious consequences for the provider.

The Boundary Around Intimate Connections: The boundary around romantic and/or sexual relationships is a very important one, and expectations for intimate partners are very different from those in other types of relationships. While intimate relationships develop in many situations, when they develop between members of a peer support group in which people are working on recovery, it can add complexity and volatility that will impact the group's work. Such relationships are common and you should watch for them in your groups. An additional layer of complexity is added when intimate relationships develop in peer support groups between people who already have other intimate relationships either inside or outside the group. For example, when intimate relations develop between group members who are already married to other people, or when intimate relations develop between members who are already intimately involved with others in the group.

The Boundary Between Participants in a Group and the Leader of the Group: While peer support group leaders are in many ways like the participants, the role of leader is different in ways that need to be maintained for the health of the group. For example, the leader is more responsible for the meetings than are the members. The leaders at times have to take actions that the members would not be expected to take. When group members or the leader act in ways that ignore that difference, it can have important negative consequences for the group. For example, when a member acts in a way that suggests that they are the leader, other members can become confused about who is ultimately responsible for the meetings.

THE VALUE OF BOUNDARIES

To understand why peer support group leaders need to pay attention to boundaries, it is important to recognize their value. Below are just a few of the key benefits of psychological boundaries.

- Boundaries reflect the shared definition of the relationships between people.
- Boundaries designate the agreed-upon degree of intimacy, and thus help create a setting in which trust and caring can develop.

- Boundaries help designate those who are responsible for something.
- Boundaries create a sense of connection between people inside the boundary.
- Boundaries can create a sense of distance from those outside the boundary.

BOUNDARY CROSSINGS

A "boundary crossing" refers to actions by one or more persons that suggest that a boundary is not present or valid. Some boundary crossings are of little importance and can be ignored. Others are more significant and will require that you as the leader respond. Below are some common examples that you will want to watch for and respond to:

- A group member violates the group expectations of confidentiality by talking about what is said in the group with outside people.
- A married group member begins having an affair with a single group member and draws other members into hiding it.
- A group member starts acting as though he is the group leader, or acts as though the leader is not the leader.
- A group member acts as though she is much closer to another member than that member is comfortable with.
- In a peer support group with closed membership, an individual who is not in the group acts as though the group is open and he can join without following the agreed-upon procedure.
- A group member talks about having a romantic relationship with her clinical provider.

STRATEGIES FOR ESTABLISHING GOOD BOUNDARIES

Many boundary crossings are caused by a lack of clarity in what is expected of people. Establishing good boundaries depends on open discussion about those boundaries. Early in the development of any peer support group, there should be some discussion of expectations, including expectations of boundaries. As leader, you will want to be sure this discussion does happen and that the group is clear about the boundaries it agrees upon.

It is important to note that some boundaries are not set by the group, but may be set by law (e.g., sexual relationships between licensed mental healthcare providers and their clients is illegal in many places) or by a sponsoring organization (e.g., a hospital may designate a group that it sponsors as a "closed group").

It is not enough to establish boundaries at the start of a group. You will want to look for opportunities to remind the group about the boundaries they have agreed upon. Such an opportunity may arise as part of reviewing a comfort agreement at the beginning of meetings, or by simply making occasional comments in the meetings, whenever necessary, to remind members of the expectations. Regardless of when or how you do it, by being explicit in your comments about boundaries, you will help members understand both the concept and why it is important to protect them.

STRATEGIES FOR RESPONDING TO BOUNDARY BREACHES

As a leader, you want to attend to actions by members or non-members that break boundaries that are important for the health of your group. It's important to note that not all boundary breaches threaten the functioning of the group, so you will not want to respond to those that are not of great risk or those that are likely to self-correct. In the case of boundary breaches that do pose a risk to the group, you will typically want to start with the least dramatic response, with the hope that a small action will be sufficient to correct the problem. If not, you will want to move on to increasingly active steps until you get the response needed. Examples of some strategies include:

- Reminding an individual member of the guidelines that the group agreed upon.
- Reminding the entire group of the guidelines that they agreed upon.
- Pointing out the breach in the group, and raising concern about its possible impact.
- Meeting a member(s) outside the group to express concern about their behaviors that break an agreed-upon boundary.
- Asking for consultation from a professional provider or other respected resource regarding how to respond to a boundary breach.

In some settings, it may be appropriate and necessary to ask a member or members to stop coming to the group if they cannot correct their behavior. This is an extreme step that is usually taken when less active steps have failed and no other option exists to correct an issue that threatens the functioning of the group.

A Final Note on Boundaries in Peer Support Groups. The concept of boundaries is often vague and confusing to those who have not heard about it before. Over time, it becomes clearer as peer support group leaders see how people act in groups and the challenges that can arise. If this concept is confusing, be patient and continue to talk with more experienced peer support group leaders to help you get a better working sense of boundaries.

CHAPTER 6

TAKING YOUR ROLE TO THE NEXT LEVEL

Basic people and organizational skills will get you started as a self-help group leader. Once you have settled into the role, your experience in leading a group will give you an opportunity to deepen those skills. Successful leaders learn from their experience, reflecting on what works and what doesn't, and changing their approach accordingly.

One thing you will learn is that the success of the group is dependent on many elements you cannot control. The members of your group will shape much of what happens in that group. Their investment, their skills and talents, their personal challenges and weaknesses, and their capacity to trust and to care about others will form much of the raw material that will determine whether your group creates a supportive environment and what the group does with that environment.

While it is only realistic to recognize that the success of the group is not dependent on you, it is still important that you learn what you can contribute, and that you seek to do your part well. Your efforts to constantly improve your contribution will result in better outcomes for the group and growth for you, both personally and in terms of skill development.

This chapter is designed to provide you with strategies you can use as you become more comfortable with the basics of leading and managing peer support groups, so that you can advance your leadership skills. We'll be working with the following assumptions:

- As previously stated, much of what happens in your group is not dependent on you or your actions. But, as the group leader/facilitator, you do have a big impact on the group and so you want to do your part well.

- Some of your job is related to the skills of facilitating meetings and shepherding both the group as a whole and the individuals in the group.

- Some of your impact depends on how you act as a member of the group. You are more visible than other members and so your words and actions will have a bigger impact on others. Members will see how you act toward others as a model for their own behavior. In addition, the way you talk about the world will help establish some of the assumptions underlying the comments made by other group members.

For these reasons, over time you will want (and need) to develop advanced skills and invest in your own personal development.

ADVANCED INTERPERSONAL SKILLS

1. <u>Understanding and Recognizing the Psychological/Social Needs of Group Members</u>. We all have a certain ability to interact with other people, though some of us have been better trained than others. Our interpersonal training has mostly been informal—in our families and our social groups. Those settings have affected, and in many cases, distorted how we understand

people and social settings. Being able to see people clearly, to recognize what they want and need, is a critical advanced skill that gives you the information you need to help the group meet its psychological/social needs. Despite our existing skills, which may already be rather advanced, there is always room for improvement.

We all need to recognize and correct some of the distortions in how we learned to see those around us. For example, our prior experiences may cause us to assume that people who look angry are going to act in aggressive ways toward others. This might lead us to try to stop people who appear to be getting angry, from talking about those feelings. This would be unfortunate, as talking about feelings of anger is one of many important things that groups can be helpful for. Similarly, our prior experience may cause us to assume that people who talk about sad feelings are going to become overwhelmed by those feelings. Again, this might lead us to try to stop people from talking openly about their disappointments and sad feelings, which would again be a lost opportunity. We typically are not aware of the distortions we have learned and so don't recognize our errors. With time and effort, we can correct those distortions, and become more accurate in understanding and responding to people's actual needs.

2. Understanding the Needs and Dynamics of Groups. Groups of people are one of the most complex and fascinating things to study and understand. While they have many predictable needs and dynamics, groups can have an infinite number of variations that the experienced leader should constantly watch for and learn from. Like individuals, groups have needs and personalities. A leader who can recognize what a group needs and how best to help it meet those needs will be able to contribute more to that group than someone who is not clear about what their group

needs. Again, we have all learned about groups informally through our own experiences in our families, in school, and in other social groups. Some of those experiences will help us as leaders, but likewise, we also have made some distorted conclusions about groups based on those experiences, and so often have some "un-learning" to do as well. For example, we may have grown up in a family in which open disagreement was avoided at all costs - in which open disagreement was seen as rebellion and betrayal of the family. People who grow up in such families often feel very uncomfortable in groups where disagreement, and even conflict, are openly discussed and worked through. A leader who grew up in such a family, may unintentionally push their group to avoid any open disagreement or conflict. This would stunt most group development, as disagreement and some conflict is a natural part of most groups.

3. <u>Understanding How to Influence Behavior—Learning About Interpersonal Interventions</u>. People come to groups often because they want something to be different in their experience. Sometimes they simply wish to feel less isolated. Quite often they join because of a number of changes that they consciously or unconsciously want to make. The group is the main tool for making those changes. As leader, your role is to help the group do its part in supporting this change.

You need to understand how people change and what groups and individuals can do to help those changes come about. By this point you know that simply giving people information about change, or encouraging them to change is often not successful. Change is complex and people are sometimes ambivalent about the changes they seek. A great deal has been written and researched in the area of how groups and individuals can help others make changes, and you will want a deepening understanding of those concepts (See the bibliography at the end of this book for several valuable resources). There are also practical skills that you will want to develop. But knowing about the skills does not mean that you have the skills, and so you will need to learn how to practice and perfect the skills so that you can have as much impact as possible. The next section explains a number of useful advanced skills that will increase your effectiveness as a leader of peer support groups.

KNOWLEDGE AND SKILLS SPECIFIC TO CERTAIN TYPES OF GROUPS

1. Understanding the Nature of the Problem or Theme That the Group Focuses On. If you are leading a group with a specific focus, you will want to know as much as possible about that focus. If you are leading a depression support group, you will need to broaden your knowledge about depression. If you are leading a support group for victims of child abuse, you will want to learn as much as you can about the impact of child abuse and domestic violence. Do not make the common mistake of thinking that your own personal experience is sufficient to understand others' experiences. Even with common experiences, there is a wide variety in what people actually go through and how they see it. For example, depression can look very different in different people. Child abuse can take many forms and people can respond in many different ways to the same form of abuse. To the degree that you understand the variations, you will be able to help the group better serve the variety of group members.

2. Understanding the Nature of Recovery/Resolution of a Problem. For those groups that focus on a problem or clinical need, you will also want to learn as much as possible about how people recover from that problem. It is not enough to know the problem well, you also need to understand the various ways that people successfully overcome or cope with it so that you can recognize and encourage the full range of positive steps in the

recovery of your group members. For example, people recover from substance-use disorders in a variety of ways. If you don't understand the range of strategies that can be helpful, you may fail to help some group members recover in a way that you are not aware of, but that may work well for them. If recovery is the goal, it's not so much *how* they get there as it is *that* they do get there. Again, don't fall into the trap of thinking that your personal recovery method is the only way—or the best way—to recover.

3. <u>Understanding the Varieties and Processes of Treatment</u>. For those groups that focus on an issue that has clinical treatments, you will want to know as much as possible about those treatments. Peer support groups work best when they complement effective clinical treatments, so a common topic in support groups is how to help members learn about and participate in these treatments. If you develop a solid knowledge of the range of available options, you can have a helpful role in making sure the group discussion reflects sound information.

4. <u>Understanding Family Dynamics</u>. For those groups that involve family members or are specific to couples, families, or parents, you will want to learn as much as you can about family dynamics. Families have their own patterns and issues that are very powerful. You want to recognize that certain issues are visible on the surface, while others lie underneath. Again, you bring your own family background with you, which can give you insight, but it can also create blinders for you as leader. Your study of family dynamics should help you understand the variety of family dynamics and experiences, while giving you more understanding of, and perspective on, your own experiences.

5. <u>Understanding Spirituality</u>. Many of the largest self-help group organizations, such as AA and other 12-step groups, have

spirituality as a central part of their model. Spirituality is a dimension of life that varies widely between people and is often not talked about openly, leaving us all with a fairly undeveloped understanding of the variety of spiritual experiences and of spiritual dynamics. If spirituality is a central part of the group you are leading, you will want to ensure you have a full understanding of the variety of spiritual experiences. You will also want to understand how to facilitate a discussion of spiritual issues in a way that communicates support for the range of people's experiences, and encourages them to speak confidently about their own experiences. This will take extra work for you, as discussions of spirituality tend to be particularly volatile, requiring active leadership to help create a firm agreement of support.

STRATEGIES FOR DEVELOPING ADVANCED KNOWLEDGE AND SKILLS

1. Take a Class. A wide range of classroom offerings can help you develop your knowledge and skills, from a single session or class to graduate coursework. You may feel that formal study is more investment than you are able or want to make. Brief classes set up for adult learning often make this an easier choice. For some leaders, the classes will contribute the deepening knowledge that they are seeking. There are a range of settings for these courses, but you may want to explore adult learning organizations and community colleges near you for some of the briefer course offerings available in your area. Online courses may be more practical for some.

2. Read. Many books and articles can be helpful in deepening your understanding and skills. If you are working in a larger organization, you will want to look for resources they provide for your development. There are a range of other materials developed by experienced clinical professionals and by

experienced peer support leaders that are appropriate for you. Pursue those that fit your need and have a format that works for you (brief articles, case studies, technical books, etc.).

3. <u>Join or Start a Support Group for Group Facilitators</u>. You may find that deepening your skills is an easier task if you do it with others. There are many peer support groups and many peer support group leaders who want advanced skills and knowledge. Look for groups of leaders who are working together to support each other's work and to help each other learn more. If there is no group near you, consider starting your own. As you know, leading a peer support group can be quite challenging, and you are likely to find a number of other group leaders who would welcome a chance to form a leadership support group.

4. <u>Get Ongoing Consultation from Experienced Group Leaders or Clinical Supervisors</u>. Individual supervision and guidance from a knowledgeable person is probably the most effective way to truly deepen your skills. Having someone review your work with you, helping you identify your successes and what you need to change, and then working with you to improve, often results in the greatest skill development. It can be a little intimidating to have someone look closely at our work, but it is worth the initial anxiety.

PERSONAL DEVELOPMENT

As noted earlier, you will have a large impact on the group because of your role as leader. How you act as a group member, how you treat others, how open you are with your thoughts and feelings, how much caring and support you show for others—all of these behaviors will set the tone for the group. Your strengths and your weaknesses will also impact the group. For this reason, continuing to pursue personal development is not only in your individual interest, but is a key way to improve your work as group leader.

You probably already recognize that being in a group, and in particular, serving as a leader of a group, gives you many opportunities for personal growth. Groups can create the caring personal connections that can lead to personal development. They can also give you an opportunity to witness your own behavior and reflect on what your feelings and actions say about who you are and how you work psychologically. Challenging experiences will often highlight both your strengths and your weaknesses, and so can frame issues that you need to work on. People avoid leadership roles for this very reason, but it actually represents a great opportunity to learn and develop as a person in ways that will pay off for you in many parts of your life. Seasoned leaders learn to value those experiences that uncover difficult truths about themselves, as this creates opportunities for growth. Some general strategies should help in this effort:

1. <u>Build Your Understanding of Yourself —Your Feelings and Your Strengths and Weaknesses</u>. The better you know and understand yourself, the more you can be of help to others. Understanding yourself will deepen your understanding and appreciation for other people and what they are experiencing. It will also increase your ability to manage your feelings and actions in a way that allows you to be better able to assist your group. The old prayer "Lord, make us masters of ourselves that we may be the servants of others" makes sense if we understand that self-understanding is the first step in self-mastery.

2. <u>Build Your Capacity to Be Known by Others—Congruence</u>. At some level, we are all looking for groups of people with whom we feel a sense of belonging and can be ourselves, including the parts of us that are similar to the group *and* the

parts that may be different. People in your group are also looking for that, even if they don't say it or are not consciously aware of it. The degree to which you are comfortable being yourself in the group sends a direct message to other members about the degree to which the group is a safe place for them to also be themselves.

"Congruence" is defined as the degree to which you act in a way that is consistent with who you really are. None of us is fully congruent all of the time, but people who are more congruent encourage others to be more congruent. Congruence is a challenge for everyone, but it is also a sign of personal development and has benefits for those around us. We all have been taught early in life about how to deal with the fact that we are similar to, and different from others. Should we hide our differences to avoid criticism? If we are open about our individual differences, how do we deal with the potentially negative way others may respond to us and the feeling of loneliness that can come with recognizing that we are each individuals?

Part of your development as a leader should include increasing your ability to let others know you as an individual—letting them see how you really think and feel about things. This will require you to find trusting relationships in which you can be yourself. It will also require you to take risks to let your differences be seen. This is a complex challenge that will take time and effort, but will help you to better model openness and self-acceptance to your group, and so will enhance your impact as a leader.

3. <u>Build Your Capacity to Be Caring Toward Others</u>. Caring is the main currency in the economy of peer support groups. Everyone wants to—and needs to—be cared about. The expectation is that peer support groups are a place where caring is exchanged. How it is exchanged and in what amounts will

depend both on how much caring group members bring to the group, and what the group's norm is for expressing caring.

As group leader, you have a direct impact on both of these factors. To the degree you have a lot of concern and interest in others, you bring caring to the group economy. As leader, the care you express tends to have a greater impact, as others naturally see your role as more important. The group will also look to you to see what the norms should be regarding caring. If they see you being generous in your support for other members, they will tend to see this as the way the group functions and will generally follow suit. If they see you being very reserved and hesitant to express support, they will again tend to follow your lead.

A word of caution about expressing caring and support. This can be done in a way that is actually counterproductive. Leaders who express caring in a way that is excessive or feels inauthentic can have a negative impact on the group, as members don't trust that the leader is expressing real feeling. Attend also to the boundaries around physical expressions of caring, since touching and hugging without permission can feel like a boundary crossing to some people.

4. <u>Build Your Capacity to Be Cared About by Others</u>. In a healthy group, members exchange caring and support. It is not healthy for this exchange to be one-sided for any extended period of time. Members need to understand the give-and-take nature of this and may come to you with challenges either in giving or receiving caring.

As leader, you need to be able to receive caring as well. I have seen many people who volunteer for leadership roles who are generous in giving support to others, but very uncomfortable receiving it. When members try to support them in any form, they bristle or look so uncomfortable that the other person feels badly. The group quickly learns that the leader is not comfortable receiving support, and some members will tend to follow this pattern.

Developing the capacity to accept caring is a challenge for some people, and often takes conscious effort to identify what feels uncomfortable about being offered support and what responses we may instinctively make to discourage or redirect expressions of caring. That knowledge, sometimes with the assistance of others, can help us change our initial reaction so that we start to be more comfortable accepting support.

5. Build Your Own Personal Resilience and Wellness Practices. The more you proactively pursue healthy disciplines that support your physical and mental wellness and build resilience to life's unexpected challenges, the more you will be able to sustain your work as a leader over time. You will also be a good model of this higher level of recovery activity for those in your group. Some of the tasks of a good self-care plan include:

- Monitoring Your Own Well-Being. To ensure that you're also tending to yourself while doing your best to help others, take note of the following tips.
  1. Ensure you know the common signs of stress, depression, and anxiety.
  2. Identify those signs that are most typical for you.
  3. Develop a plan for how to respond to problems before they develop.
- Committing to Healthy Living. A number of lifestyle factors are associated with positive mental health and build resilience for those working in stressful roles (like peer support group leader). Those with clear research support include:

1. Eating a healthy diet.
2. Maintaining a healthy weight.
3. Exercising regularly.
4. Maintaining a good sleep routine.
5. Maintaining good social support and healthy relationships.
6. Making sure that fun is a regular part of your life.
7. Avoiding smoking.
8. Learning to relax and manage stress.
9. Practicing some form of spirituality.
10. Offering contribution and service to others (i.e., altruism).

STRATEGIES FOR ENHANCING YOUR OWN PERSONAL DEVELOPMENT

There are a number of practical strategies that people use to support their own personal development. Consider adopting some of the following:

- Journaling. Gaining self-awareness of your own feelings and actions is one of the key elements of personal development. Self-awareness will help you recognize and improve what you are doing in groups. It will also sharpen your recognition of your own feelings, which often are a valuable source of information about what is happening in the group at a deeper level. A fairly simple strategy that will build your self-awareness is to spend some time each day writing in a journal about your daily experience. It can be difficult at first to find the time to develop this routine, but once started, the benefits of journaling will likely keep you using this simple strategy.

- Friends Who Will Be Honest with You. Everyone needs people in their lives who care about them enough, or are courageous enough, to give them honest feedback. We all have blind spots, and the most common way to see them is with the help of those who care about us. You will want to be proactive in developing those types of relationships— encourage frank feedback from those around you and reward those who give it to you.

- Expand Supportive Personal Relationships. As healthy soil and water are to plants, so supportive relationships are to people—they help us grow. A large body of research highlights the key role that supportive relationships play in almost every part of healthy living. Consciously working at building your network of supportive friends is a simple strategy that will naturally lead to personal growth.

- Set Goals for Congruence, Caring, and Wellness Practices. Consciously planning how you will become more congruent, more caring toward others, and more engaged in those behaviors that encourage physical and emotional wellness will lead to personal growth. You may not meet all of your goals, but the fact that you set specific goals and think about how to achieve them will lead you to move toward them.

- Individual Psychotherapy. Some people find that individual psychotherapy is a key to getting significant momentum in personal growth and development. This may be particularly helpful in working through emotional challenges that are not getting resolved by less intensive methods.

CHAPTER 7

HOW DO PEER SUPPORT GROUPS INTERFACE WITH FORMAL CARE SERVICES?

Some voices in the healthcare community have wondered whether peer support groups compete with formal (professional) care services, or could even replace some types of formal care in a way that would save healthcare dollars. The available data suggests that this is not the case. People who attend peer support groups are more likely to also be receiving formal care, suggesting that they see the combination of peer and formal support as better than either service used alone. Other research studies suggest that these people are correct—the combination of formal care and participation in peer support groups is associated with better outcomes (see appendix A).

Peer support groups are natural partners to formal care providers. They provide attendees with information that can help them be better patients and better consumers of formal care services. Peer support groups also provide encouragement and support to attendees, who then tend to remain in care longer, in a way that usually results in better clinical outcomes. In addition, these groups often help attendees transition successfully out of formal care by providing the social support needed to make that transition. From this perspective, peer support groups are complementary to—not a substitute for—formal care, often addressing needs that clinical providers cannot address.

Providers, however, do not always see peer support groups as partners. Many are simply unaware of the large number and type of groups available to their patients or even that their patients are attending such groups. Because peer support groups give attendees access to practical information about formal care, including specific information about experiences with different providers, some providers feel threatened by their potential influence. This concern can be reasonable when the provider is worried about potential misinformation being spread by well-intentioned but uneducated consumers. But it can be unreasonable when the provider is concerned that the sharing of accurate information may result in some consumers not choosing to use their services or being more informed and/or more assertive consumers. A natural tension exists in the relationship between peer support groups and formal providers that represents the realistic potential for peer support groups to provide accurate or inaccurate information to attendees. This relationship is likely to evolve as peer support group leaders learn to ensure that group meetings provide accurate information, and as providers learn more about the benefits of peer support groups and collaborate more with them.

PEER SUPPORT GROUPS AND THE PHASES OF FORMAL CARE

The natural partnership between formal providers and peer support groups changes in focus over the course of treatment.

<u>Outreach and Pre-Treatment</u>. For a great deal of medical care, there is a delay between the time individuals need care and when they actually begin to receive it. This is particularly true in the case of mental health care, where the delays are often years in length.

Delays can be costly, as additional problems often accrue as a result of untreated healthcare needs. The reasons for these delays are complex and vary by person and condition. While the temptation is to look for external barriers to people entering care (e.g. insurance, wait times for appointments), most of the research data points to significant internal barriers to people choosing to enter care: internalized stigma, anxiety about admitting to having a need, the desire to deal with the problem independently. These barriers are often related to the lack of recognition of a need, lack of understanding about how to enter care, or lack of willingness to seek help. The result is that a large number of people who have clinical needs are not in treatment.

Peer support groups have a potentially key role in addressing this situation. Many people who are ambivalent about entering formal care may feel more willing to attend a peer support group. Family members and friends may find it easier to convince their relatives and friends to attend a peer group, as opposed to a doctor's appointment. For these and other reasons, it is possible, even probable, that some people will come to peer support groups as the first step in entering formal care. In that situation, peer support groups can provide some key resources:

- Basic information about the problem, treatment, and recovery.
- Basic information about the personal experience of the illness and recovery.
- Encouragement and support for recognizing and taking action to get treatment for a problem.

- Support and information about entering and participating in formal care.

Early Care. People who are in early phases of treatment for most significant physical or mental health issues have some common needs, some of which can be met by formal providers, but some of which can be met in complementary ways by peer support groups. They include needs for:

- Information about the illness and the future experience of the illness, e.g., how does the experience of the illness change over time, what is the prognosis, what is recovery like, what might help.
- Information about common forms of care, local providers, and practical guidelines about how to navigate early care.
- Information about common mistakes or potential dead-ends in care, and how to avoid them.
- Encouragement not to stop treatment early.

The Middle Phase of Care. People in the middle phase of care have often learned a great deal about treatment and what works for them. They have ongoing relationships with formal providers, but may need help making ongoing decisions about care. Peer support groups can address a number of these needs, including:

- Information about additional treatment options and the personal experience other members have had with the treatment and the providers.
- Information about the experience of care during this phase.
- In some cases, the focus of ongoing care shifts from formal providers to the person with the illness. For example, illnesses like diabetes require ongoing patient disease self-management. Peer groups can provide an

opportunity to share the experience of independent self-management.

- Opportunities to give back to others by sharing what they have learned through their illness. This aspect is a highly valued element of attending peer support groups, and those who can find a way to turn their often painful struggles with an illness into a benefit to others often feel that there has been some redeeming aspect of the illness.

Discharge and Post-Care. As people transition out of formal care, peer support groups can address a range of important needs, including:

- Support for the discharge process, which can be difficult for some. This can take the form of sharing information or providing emotional support for the process of leaving formal care, or simply interacting with people who have successfully transitioned out of care.
- Additional support for disease self-management, which may continue for many illnesses after formal care has ended.
- The need for ongoing or transitional social support from a community that knows the experience of the illness and recovery.
- The opportunity to give back to others through peer support opportunities.

MAXIMIZING THE BENEFITS OF COLLABORATION BETWEEN FORMAL CARE AND PEER SUPPORT GROUPS

While some peer support groups work closely with formal care providers, and may even be developed and supported within healthcare organizations, most are not. A number of peer support organizations purposely do not communicate with healthcare providers—it is important that you know and follow the guidelines of your group regarding this issue. When communication and collaboration are possible, a few strategies are key to maximizing the benefit for participants.

<u>Maintain Good Communication Between Formal Care and Peer Support</u>. The natural partnership between peer support groups and formal healthcare providers works most effectively when there is adequate communication. Communication may be helpful when:

- Formal care providers need to know what peer support groups are available to the patients they serve.
- Formal care providers need to refer patients to relevant groups.
- Peer support group members need referral to appropriate providers.
- Peer support groups and providers have developed a close collaboration, including permissions from participants to communicate about ongoing participation.
- Peer support leaders would like consultation and/or ongoing supervision from appropriate providers.
- Peer support group members appear to be in such a severe crisis that they need emergency help from formal care providers.

It is important to note that *good* communication does not mean a *large amount* of communication. Most participants in peer support groups do not desire that their comments in the group be communicated to their healthcare providers. Instead, they value the opportunity to talk openly in an uncensored way.

To protect this aspect of the group experience, it is important that communication with providers be limited to a few topics that participants understand and approve of beforehand. The most valuable topics may include (1) information needed to refer someone to the group or from the group to formal care, (2) ongoing attendance, (3) evidence of the person being in crisis, and (4) evidence of the person needing a change in the formal care he or she is receiving.

Coordination of Efforts. Collaboration between peer support groups and formal care providers is possible when a few strategies are followed.

- Participants must first want to collaborate. Group members must see the benefit of communication between peer support groups and formal care before they are willing to support it. Communication will require permission in the form of signed consent for each party to communicate with another party. If you have limited experience with these legal permissions, speak with your supervisor or with the formal care providers about this.

- Both the peer support group leaders and the formal providers should know of each other's work and agree on some level of collaboration in order to better help the people they both serve. This may take some effort by one or more parties to educate the other about what they do and how collaboration can benefit patients.

- Both group leaders and formal providers should have clear expectations of what will be communicated and when.

REFERRALS FROM HEALTHCARE PROVIDERS TO PEER SUPPORT GROUPS

It is in the interest of many healthcare providers to develop a network of peer support groups to which they can routinely refer patients. Peer support groups provide additional services and support that many patients need, and so the health of those patients will be improved if they participate in groups in addition to formal care. Some providers will understand this synergy and others will not. Research studies cited in appendix A can help you to show providers that in many cases, it is in their patients' interest to be referred to peer support groups.

Healthcare providers can refer their patients to peer support groups in various ways. Research suggests that many people need strong encouragement to join a group if they are to do so. Some of the practices that have been shown to be most successful include the following steps:

- The provider directly recommends to the patient that he attend a peer support group.
- The provider gives the patient a handout describing available groups, including the date/time of meetings, as well as the location, with directions.
- The provider asks the patient for their perception of the pros and cons for attending the group(s) and discusses them.
- The provider discusses with the patient what meetings are like and what is expected of participants.
- The provider has a peer support group member meet with the patient to introduce herself, talk about why she attends, and arrange to meet the patient at the meeting. If necessary, the member may provide transportation to the meeting.
- The provider gets permission to share the patient's phone number with a peer support group facilitator who will call and invite the patient, giving information about attendance.
- The provider follows up with the patient at a later appointment, checking to see if he attended and if not, encourages him to do so.

Many providers will not be willing to use all of these steps, but those who recognize the benefits for their patients will be interested in finding the most effective ways of encouraging them to join a group.

REFERRALS FROM PEER SUPPORT GROUPS TO HEALTHCARE PROVIDERS

Over the course of your work facilitating peer support groups, you are going to come across group members who need additional clinical care but don't know how to find it. You can be very helpful in referring them to an appropriate provider. Experienced peer group leaders maintain a list of providers whom they can refer members to, and they carry contact information for these providers with them to give to interested people. The final chapter of this book provides you a simple format for recording contact information for providers. Take the time to review that table and fill out the information for those providers you know of at this time. Over time, you are likely to hear about others whom group members like to work with. Add their information to your list, as you will need a growing resource list for the range of people you will support with referrals.

WHEN AND HOW TO COMMUNICATE

In general, you will want to work this out with the provider. Arrangements vary widely depending on the situation and personal preferences. Recognize the following:

- There are legal restrictions regarding the communication of healthcare information. The provider will likely know more about these than you, and can help you ensure your communication follows the rules. You will want to learn about them as well.
- Healthcare providers are generally very busy and so communication will need to be limited if they are going

to be able to participate. Be attentive to what they can and want to do in terms of communication and be respectful of the demands they are facing.

- When communicating about a crisis, be aware that they will need basic information so that they can take quick action. If possible, be ready with the basic information they will need, including the name and location of the person, the concern you have, and the evidence that causes you to be concerned.

POTENTIAL PROBLEMS

Collaboration between formal providers and peer support group leaders does have some risks that are worth noting.

- The participant may be confused as to what is formal care and what is peer support. Participants in peer support groups may not understand that the group and the group leaders are not part of their formal care or they may misunderstand what kind of care they are receiving.
- Peer support group leaders may feel pressure from those providers they collaborate with, particularly in regard to agendas other than the support of their patients. For example, providers may be interested in collaborating as a means of getting new patients, or of discharging patients they don't want to see. They may also want the peer support group to encourage treatment compliance.

Open communication and recognition/acceptance of the different agendas of peer support groups and formal care are two key strategies for dealing with these dangers. If you are collaborating with formal care providers or are interested in exploring collaboration, you will want to talk about these potential dangers with your peers and/or supervisor.

CHAPTER 8

FORMING A NEW GROUP

Forming a new group is often more difficult than you might expect. Many groups don't make it, which is painful and can have negative consequences. A common scenario is that only a few people come to the first few meetings. Potential attendees come, see a small number of other people and as a result, feel concerned that there must be something wrong with the group ("Why doesn't anyone want to come to this group -- must be something wrong with it"), and don't return. Other times it is less clear why a group never really gets off the ground. In most situations, groups that have trouble forming, do so because there was not adequate preparation work. If you plan to start a new group, you'll want to think about the following strategies.

LOOK FOR PARTNERS

Starting a new group often takes work that is better done by a group than an individual. If you can, look for partners who want to help get the group started. They can help with the tasks that will be required, and their opinions and suggestions will help in the planning.

IDENTIFYING A NEED

A key determinant of whether a new group will succeed, is whether the group meets a need that people feel. The need has to include the focus of the group (e.g. supporting sobriety, providing information about pregnancy, providing support after the loss of a loved one) but also has to address other factors (e.g. "I need a group in the evening", "I need a group I can reach with public transportation", "I need a group where I feel comfortable being a teenager").

Sometimes the needs are so obvious that it takes little effort to be confident that we know what they are. More often, we may feel like we know, but we may not. Some simple strategies that can help ensure that you know the real need that will support a new group include the following:

1. <u>Consider Doing A Simple Survey Of The Needs and Preferences Of Potential Attendees.</u> This can be a short basic survey that can be distributed to likely groups of attendees. You may need to work with partners to get help distributing the survey to people who might use the group (e.g. get healthcare providers to distribute it to those in treatment). You may also be able to get help constructing the survey and tabulating the results.

2. <u>Consider Asking Attendees Of Other Peer Support Groups What Needs For New Groups They Are Aware Of.</u> Those already using peer support groups often know what unmet needs exist. Remember not to only ask about the focus of the group, but also about the time, location, and target population (e.g. women, young people, families)

3. <u>Ask Informal Opinion Leaders.</u> There are usually informal leaders among the attendees of peer support groups. They are often in touch with a large number of potential attendees and

know the trends in what people are saying and thinking. Consider asking these individuals for a chance to talk and then collect their input about what needs they see.

4. <u>Consider Asking Formal Providers What Needs For Additional Groups They Are Aware Of</u>. They may be very aware of groups of patients who would be willing to attend a group but can't find one that has the right focus, time, location, etc.

CREATING A FOCUS/MISSION

Once you have identified a need or needs that the group will hopefully help address, you and your partners should try to create a clear focus or mission for the new group. This is a simple sentence that summarizes what the group will provide and how it will help. It may be as simple as "the new group will extend the local 12-step groups to Tuesday evenings". It may also be more complex, such as "the new group will provide peer support to parents of disabled children, who need support that they can receive in the evenings paired with volunteer child-care". The key to a good mission statement is that it is short, focused, and captures all of the key elements of what the group will provide.

SELECTING A TIME AND PLACE

Many new groups do not survive because the time is inconvenient or the place is poorly suited for the group. You will want input on appropriate times, and possible places. Let potential members, and even early attenders help finalize a good day and time for the group. The location may be more challenging, as there are often limited options. Be attentive to issues such as size of space, cleanliness and comfort of the space, amount and ease of parking, and access for possible members who need wheelchair access. Some spaces that are commonly used (churches, schools, etc.) may have associations that some potential members will not feel comfortable with. For example, some attendees may have strong feelings about going to the building of a religious organization. Other potential sites might have formal restrictions on use of their space. For example, some organizations may require liability insurance for self-help groups that want to use their space.

RECRUITING A STARTING CORE OF ATTENDEES

As previously noted, the beginning of a new group is often a tricky phase. For a healthy beginning, a group needs to start with enough attendees so that people who come will see that the group is viable. Potential members who come to a first meeting are almost always asking a few common questions:

- Is this group something that will benefit me?
- Does this group look safe - physically and emotionally safe? Might I get criticized or treated poorly in this group? Is there some sense of structure and leadership among the members that will ensure I and others are safe?
- Is the group big enough that I will be comfortable (many people find groups of less than 5 people uncomfortable, though this can vary depending on expectations).
- Is the group small enough that I will get to talk (many people feel that groups of more than 15 are "too large", though this again varies, depending on expectations).
- Are there other people in the group that I will learn something from -- people who may be further along in their recovery, more experienced in the area of interest, etc.

Once a group is meeting regularly, it is often easier for potential members to see that the group has enough members and has something for them. In the beginning, this can be more difficult. You may want to consider setting up the first 4-8 meetings so that any potential members attending will see at least 5 attendees, at least some of whom are fairly advanced in their experience in recovery (or whatever the focus of the group is) and experienced in being in a peer support group. Experienced group members (sometimes called "ringers") will help to establish good group norms from the beginning and will enrich the discussion with a more seasoned perspective.

It may be worth considering having a professional clinician as a co-leader in the first 4-8 sessions, again to help establish the norms of the group and help create a sense of safety for those coming for the first time. Once a group is established, any professional leader and any invited "ringer" may want to stop coming, as the group is more likely to function well and will be seen as a more established safe place to prospective visitors.

CONNECTING WITH FORMAL CARE ORGANIZATIONS AND OTHER POTENTIAL REFERRAL SOURCES

There are a number of community organizations that will want to know about your group, depending on the focus. These organizations include local health care organizations and professionals, social service organizations, employee assistance counselors, members of the clergy, and school counselors and courts.

There are many reasons for considering talking with them about your plans to start a new group.
- They can provide information about the need for a new group.

- They can provide referrals to the group.
- They can sometimes provide space for the group.
- If they have patients who may want to attend the group, you may need to start or expand your partnership with them around those attendees.

If you have an existing relationship with a provider or organization, it is easy enough to let them know about your interest in starting a new group. If you don't have an existing relationship, you'll need to do a little more work. Consider the following steps:

- Look for sources of information about the provider and the potential for talking with them about a new self-help group. You may want to try to find out which individual in an organization may be the best candidate for working with you.
- Ask for a chance to talk with them about the new group. Explain who you are, what you are interested in doing, why it is related to their work, and how they could help. For example, something like the following might be a good way to start the conversation.

  "Hi Dr. Johnson. My name is xxxx, and I am one of the facilitators for the new mothers' support group across the street on Tuesday mornings. Many of your patients attend this group and it is going very well. We are considering starting a new group in the evening to help those who can't attend during the day, and I wonder if you might have 15 minutes sometime soon when we could talk about this new group. I could use your help getting the word out about it."

- When you do get a chance to talk, be respectful of their time. Be clear about what you are doing and what you are asking of them. Look for ways to partner with them and ways they may benefit from the group. Be clear in what you ask them and ask of them.

- Follow-up on any items you commit to, and give them updates as part of your follow-up (e.g. "Dr. Johnson, I just wanted to follow-up on our meeting from last month. We did start that group and there are about 5 mothers attending every Tuesday evening. Let me know if I can provide you or your patients with any more information about the group. We'd love to have your support letting potential members know about it.")

CONSIDER FINDING A CONSULTANT

Many group leaders have a more experienced leader, or a healthcare professional, that they use as an outside consultant to help them in their role. You may have situations in the group in which you are not sure what is going on or what your response should be. Having an experienced consultant to talk with between meetings, and who can help you develop your own skills and insights, will be a great resource for you. Finding the right person for you typically takes some effort. Consider people who are running similar groups, who are working in related clinical fields, or who other group leaders have used as consultants or mentors in the past. In some settings, clinical providers who refer their patients to the groups may be willing to provide consultation as part of supporting your work.

PUBLICIZING THE GROUP

Any strategy to publicize a new group has to start with the goal of the group. What is the mission of the group and what is the target population that it will serve. Publicity should be designed to inform that target population about the group with a message that both attracts their attention, and tells them the basics of the group (what, where, when). Strategizing about the publicity for a group often takes more thought than most new group leaders recognize, but if you want a group to start well, it is worth the time and effort.

Again, an effective notice must be brief and clear. It often has some wording or image to get people's attention. Common strategies for getting people's attention include:

- Start with a question(s) (e.g. "Are you a new parent? Would you like a chance to connect with other new parents and share support and information?)

- Start with a provocative statement or curious (Parenting is the most important skill that we are never taught!)

- Start with a humorous statement ("Do you change diapers in your sleep?").

- If you are creating a visual notice like a flyer or web-based notice, consider using unusual, colorful, and eye-catching graphics to get people's attention.

While it is often valuable to create notices and flyers, most people who come to a peer support/self-help group will come because of a personal contact -- someone they know who tells them to come to the group or invites them to come to the group. Group members, including those people who are planning on attending a new group, will often be the most effective source for recruiting new members. You will want to remind members of that fact and encourage them to think of who they could invite, and to give personal invitations. Other people to notify as to new groups include:

- Local social service agencies
- Local community resources (town officials, clergy, public health officials, etc.)
- Peer Specialists
- Other peer support groups/self-help groups

- Local print, TV and radio resources, such as a town newspaper, a local access TV or radio show related to health or wellness

Common Places To Post Notices

- National and/or regional web-based listings of peer support groups by agency (for example, many 12-step programs have their own directory of group meeting times and locations. See Chapter 15 for a sampling of lists).
- Local programs, clinical offices
- Local social service agencies
- Hospitals
- Libraries
- Local public access TV stations
- Town and local websites

HOLDING THE FIRST MEETING

The first meeting for a new group is particularly important for setting the tone for how the group will function. As noted before, you will want to work hard to ensure that at least five people will be at the first meeting. You may also want to ensure there are several attendees who are experienced in participating in peer support groups and are invested in helping this new group get started. Talk with them before the first meeting to help them see that they have a special role in getting the group going. You may want to consider a few other steps for the first meeting.

1. Show Up Early And Get The Physical Setting Organized.
Prospective members will be looking at the physical setting to see if they are going to be comfortable. Preparing the setting

communicates that you are invested in serving the group and that you are organized and conscientious.

2. Welcome Attendees. Assume that many of the people coming to the first meeting will be feeling a little uncertain about the group -- probably a little nervous. You may feel nervous as well, but you want to appear to be calm, warm and friendly. This starts with offering a friendly welcome to those showing up so that they know that you as the leader, are glad they are there.

3. Introducing the Group. As the leader it will probably fall to you to make an opening statement introducing the group. You will want to state the mission of the group, why it was started and possibly a brief background of how it started. If other people in the room had a part in the set-up of the group, be sure to acknowledge them.

4. Inviting Ownership of the Group. Your opening statement, and possibly other comments in this first meeting, should explicitly ask the members to join you in "owning" or taking responsibility for the group. This needs to be genuine, as the members are the owners of a group. You want this to be an invitation, recognizing that some will be happy to join you in taking responsibility, while others may be more ambivalent.

5. Framing the Start. It is often helpful to remind those attending the first few meetings of a new group, that the experience of a new group is a little different from an established group, and that the group has some work to do to get started. This "framing" of the start will help remind people that they should have different expectations for these first few meetings and they need to make extra effort to ensure it goes well.

6. Developing a Comfort Agreement. You will want to ask the group to establish an initial agreement about the basic guidelines of group meetings. A sample set of guidelines, sometimes called a "comfort agreement", can be found in chapter 8. Having the group set this up from the beginning is another way to encourage a sense of ownership, and underlines the importance of good behavior during meetings -- reassuring members that this will be a safe place to be.

7. Starting To Work. The first meeting should not be spent entirely talking about setting up the group. It is usually important for people to talk about themselves and to engage in the type of peer support that they are looking for from the group as it goes forward.

8. Closing the First Meeting. It is often useful to check-in with attendees in the last 10 minutes of the first group to see how they are feeling about the meeting. You can mention that since this is the first group, you wanted to spend just a little time at the end to see what their experience of the group was, including things they liked and things they might want to see change. This will again encourage ownership of the group by the members, while giving you an indication of what they enjoyed and whether they are likely to come back next time. If reasonable suggestions for are made, you will want to take quick action on those to show that you are responsive their needs.

BUILDING THE GROUP OVER TIME

Building a healthy group will take time and effort. If you have correctly identified a need that a significant number of people have for the group, then building the group involves helping people find out about something that they need. Your task is to help publicize the group effectively.

Most groups of people will have to deal with people leaving and new people coming. Some new group leaders have difficulty with people leaving the group, feeling that this somehow reflects on their ability to lead the group, indicating some type of failure. It is much more likely that people leave because of one of three factors: (1) the many factors in other parts of their lives are changing and shifting (work, family, duties), causing them to have to change their plans; (2) a mismatch between the person's needs and preferences and those of the rest of the group; or (3) the basic ambivalence the person feels toward openly talking about the issue or getting help for the issue. As a leader, these factors are not directly in your control and you will <u>not</u> want to take it personally when people leave.

The exception to this recommendation is when you have feedback that there is something you are doing as leader that may be contributing to people leaving. Sometimes people who are leaving a group will offer this feedback to you as part of saying goodbye. Again, new leaders sometimes take offense or feel hurt when leaving members mention something that could have been better about the group. Experienced leaders know that such feedback is a valuable gift, and actually ask people who are leaving to give them feedback about how the group could be better. It is that type of feedback that can help you continue to improve your leadership skills and thus, make the group more effective.

Assuming that your group is like almost every other peer support group, you'll need to keep an eye on the number of people joining the group to ensure that the size of the group does not shrink to a point that threatens the effectiveness. You will want to have a set of strategies that you can use to recruit new members. They typically look like the strategies suggested earlier in this chapter to recruit the original members. Many groups keep up some continuous recruitment efforts, such as keeping invitations to the group in local print sources (web-sites, local papers, religious institution bulletins, etc.). Others keep an on-going partnership with clinical providers who refer a steady flow of their patients to the group.

You will want to think about what you will do if the group grows to a point that you feel may be a problem. This depends on the nature of the group and the preferences of the members. When groups get beyond 12-15 attendees, the discussion can change in nature, resulting in less time per person for comments. Larger groups have some valuable qualities (see Chapter 12), but they are different than smaller groups. If you want to limit the size of the group, you may want to consider a few common strategies:

- Bring the topic of the size of the group up in the meeting in order to give members a chance to talk about their feelings about it, their preferences, and what steps the group wants to take.
- Consider stopping all recruitment strategies when the group reaches the target size.
- Consider adding a meeting of the group so that individual meetings will be smaller but the group will remain intact.
- Consider splitting the group. Let the group talk about how to do this in a way that creates two new healthy groups.
- Consider letting the natural impact of the larger membership level out the size of the group. For many groups, when the size of the group becomes too large, new members will stop joining because the group will not be as attractive. The danger of this strategy is that the group may not level off, or it may level off at a size that still feels too large to the members.

CHAPTER 9

ENDING A GROUP

The leadership role is very important during the process of ending a group. Ending tends to be difficult regardless of whether the group was time-limited and so everyone knew the group was going to end, or whether the group did not have a scheduled end, but instead decided to end or circumstances made it clear that they needed to end. If group members have connected to each other, saying goodbye will be a challenging task that some will find difficult. Without thoughtful leadership, many groups will end in a way that leaves a lot of important thoughts and feelings unspoken. Done well, an ending of a group can be of great help to the members, and can enhance their feelings about participating in the group, and the positive memories they keep about the group.

In thinking about how to end a group, it is important to assume that many members will have ambivalent feelings about ending. They likely recognize the need to end. They may also feel some relief about ending, either because they may feel some vulnerability sharing with the group or because they feel some frustration or challenges caused by the group. At the same time, they will likely feel sadness about ending the group, anticipating the loss of connection to the other members, and the loss of the opportunity to share themselves and be supported. Often their feelings are connected to other experiences of endings -- ending other important relationships and ending participation in other valued groups. Some of the emotions related to ending groups are related to this common association to other goodbyes.

Some people have particular problems with ending relationships and saying goodbyes. Their emotional reactions are so strong that their actions around the ending will be important for you to attend to as leader. Sometimes, they will try to leave the group before the group actually ends. This is typically an effort to avoid the feeling of saying goodbye by preemptively leaving. Sometimes they will fight the effort to end the group, actively arguing that the group should not end, even when it is clear that the group needs to end. Sometimes they will just become more distant from the group, saying less and attending less. All of these responses are signs that the person is having some difficulty coping with their feelings about ending the group.

In general, healthy groups deal with the task of ending by talking about the experience, saying goodbye, and possibly doing something to create a memory or legacy to honor their experience of the group. These are direct ways to deal with the loss of the group. As leader, you want to encourage these strategies. When you notice the group or individual members having trouble saying goodbye, you will want to help redirect them toward more healthy ways of saying goodbye.

As leader, you will want to help the group to consider a few key factors related to ending.

WHEN TO END

Some groups are time-limited and so members know from the beginning when the end will take place. For others, the decision to end will include the need to set a date. This is the group's decision, but be aware that many groups will show their ambivalence about ending by struggling with the task of setting an end date. As leader, you can often be helpful by pointing out the group's struggle with this fairly simple task, and encouraging the members to talk about their feelings while being decisive about a date.

TALKING ABOUT THE END

As noted above, it is safe assumption that most group members will have feelings about ending the group that will be important to talk about. As leader, the group is likely to need you to help them do this talking. The most common sign that they need your help is that they do not talk about ending despite the end of the group approaching. As leader, you want to point out the group's avoidance of this topic. This is a way to encourage them to reflect on why they are avoiding, but also to encourage them to start talking about saying goodbye. Some possible ways to encourage this discussion include:

- Asking members to be active in the process of deciding to end, when to end.
- Once the end date is set, reminding members at each meeting about the end date and invite their thoughts about it. You may feel some resistance to talking about this topic, and some irritation pointed at you for mentioning the topic. That is often a good sign that you are effectively pushing an important topic.
- Raise the topic of how people cope with endings. Present this as a common challenge that many people struggle with -- this will help people to feel more comfortable sharing any struggles they are feeling.

- Raise the topic of what members will be doing after the end to make up for the loss of the group.
- Raise the topic of how members will remember the group after it is over.
- Raise the topic of whether the group wants to do something special for their last meeting -- going to dinner, holding the meeting in a special place, doing something to help commemorate the group or create a shared memory.

DEALING WITH COMMON CHALLENGES

As noted, there are some common behaviors by group members that signal that they are struggling with the group ending. They include:

- The member who fights the ending of the group.
- The member who wants to avoid talking about the end.
- The member who tries to leave early, either missing more meetings, or finding a reason to stop coming entirely.
- The member who tries to create a replacement group to avoid saying goodbye.

These behaviors can actually damage the natural process of ending the group, leaving the group with a more negative memory of their experience together. For this reason, group leaders need to be vigilant for these behaviors and respond fairly quickly. Some common strategies to deal with any of these behaviors include:

- During a meeting, inviting general discussion about the topic of saying goodbye and invite members to check-in with how they are coping with saying goodbye.
- During a meeting(s), point out the efforts of individual members to fight ending and invite the group to reflect on why they may not want to end the group.

- Meet individually with members who are struggling with ending, helping them to talk about their feelings in a more focused manner.

- In extreme situations, encourage the member to talk about their feelings of ending with other professional providers they may have (e.g. their psychotherapist).

THE LAST SESSION

All of the issues that members feel about saying goodbye will be most prominent at the last session. Because it is the last meeting, the memory of what happens at this session often is one of the most powerful for members, lasting long after the group is over. For this reason, the last session is particularly important for the leader to manage. Your goal is to have the meeting be an opportunity to again talk about the ending of the group, what the group has meant to members, and then to end the meeting (and the group) in a way that leaves a positive memory of the entire group. This will be different for each group but you as leader will need to be active to ensure that the final meeting ends smoothly.

CHAPTER 10

DEALING WITH "DIFFICULT" GROUP MEMBERS

Part of the challenge of helping a peer support group achieve the healthy functioning described in chapter 2, is that some members will have patterns of behavior that take away from the group experience. This is very predictable, and the behaviors fall into such common patterns that the experienced leader will have had plenty of opportunities to learn how to effectively deal with them.

It is important to realize that in most cases, these individuals are not disrupting the group process on purpose. Their behavior usually represents their effort to deal with their own feelings about being in a group. Often the patterns of behavior have a long history for that person, and may have undermined their participation in other groups. They want to connect with others in a healthy collaborative way, but may need help in doing so.

While some of these difficult behaviors are so extreme that they should be dealt with primarily in an individual clinical setting with a mental health professional, most are not - and can be dealt with effectively by you as the group leader. The key tasks are:

(1) to recognize the pattern, (2) to understand what the behavior is seeking to achieve and to use that understanding to maintain a caring stance toward the person, and (3) to take steps to help the person change their behavior in order to get what they want while allowing the group to function in a healthier manner.

Taking action is the critical responsibility for the leader. While some mild challenges will resolve themselves, many will actually get worse, creating a great deal of tension in the group that can threaten the willingness of other group members to continue. You will want to think about a hierarchy of possible actions you can take to correct a problem behavior.

Your first possible steps should be simple actions that would correct the effects of the behavior in the group, encouraging the member and/or the group to recognize the problem behavior. If the behavior does not respond to simple actions on your part, you may have to escalate your efforts. Moderate level actions include steps such as pointing out patterns in the problem behavior to the group, asking the group to talk about their feelings about the pattern of behavior, asking members to talk about how the behaviors impact their feelings about attending the group. If these steps don't achieve any change, you may want to speak with the individual outside the group meeting to point out the behavior and its effect on the group, and to express your concern as facilitator.

In some cases, these actions will not change the behavior. If the behavior is severe enough that it threatens the group, you may have to be even more forceful, meeting with the person for a formal meeting outside the group, asking them for specific changes in their behavior, suggesting that they may need to take a break from the group, or even asking that they stop coming to the group. If you have any supervisors or consultants helping you in your role, you will want to work closely with them on these tricky situations. You may also want to draw them in to help you deal with the person.

Let's review several of the most common patterns.

THE DOMINATING VOICE

In a peer support group, the amount of meeting time in which members are talking is usually distributed fairly evenly between members, at least over the course of several meetings. Part of participation is spending time both sharing and listening.

Some members may not be attentive to this basic economy of sharing time. They take more time sharing their feelings with the group and seem unaware that this violates the basic assumption of equal sharing of attention and support. They may be quick to start talking at the beginning of the group, quick to jump in to respond to others' comments, and quick to change topics. They take up more than their share of the group's time.

They may also dominate in the way they talk to the group. Their comments may imply that they know what everyone else should do, that they have already experienced what others are going through and so have advice that everyone should follow. Regardless of whether they in fact have good advice, talking in a way that implies others should listen to them is typically experienced as disrespect by the other members.

There are several reasons why people may tend toward acting like a "dominating voice". Some people feel a deep hunger for attention from others, and so jump to take advantage of the group meeting. Often the person has poor insight into their behavior -- they do not keep track of how much time they are taking in the meeting, they do not recognize how others respond to their domination of the discussion. Sometimes, the tendency to dominate the discussion reflects the person's need to have some control in their lives, and an open discussion about problems that may not be solved, triggers their feelings that life is not in control.

Regardless of their reason, the "dominating voice" must learn to (1) share time fairly evenly with other group members and (2) comment in a way that reflects respect for the autonomy of the other members.

Examples of initial comments you could make to help this happen include:

- We've heard a lot from you tonight, John. I wonder how others are doing.
- How are we doing tonight as far as evenly sharing the discussion? Does everyone feel they are getting a chance to be heard?

The next level of comments might include:

- John, I've noticed that you have spoken more than anyone else for the last 4 meetings. What do you think about that?
- We've been talking about John speaking so often in every group. I wonder how other members feel about this. Does it have any impact on how you feel about coming to the group?

Advanced comments are often made during an individual meeting with the member outside the group. These comments might include:

- John, I think we need to come to an agreement about how much you and other members talk. I understand that you want to share a lot with the group, but for the sake of the other members, we need a clear way to ensure the time is shared more evenly. Would you be willing to agree to limit your own comments to xxxx time?

- John, we've been talking for some time now about your tendency to dominate the group discussion. Several members are very concerned that you've not changed this behavior despite their requests and my requests. What do you think needs to happen in order for this to be corrected?

- John, we've been talking about your tendency to dominate the group for some time now. Several members are very concerned that you've not changed this behavior despite their requests and my requests. Given all that we've tried in order fix this, I think it might be best if you take a break from attending the group for a while. That would give the group a break, and could give you a chance to think about this issue. If in the future, you feel more able to participate as a group member, you and I could sit down and talk about that.

THE SILENT MEMBER

In one sense, the "silent member" is the counterpart of the dominating member. They tend not to share or they share very little, failing to take part like other members. When they do make comments, the comments may reveal relatively little about them.

Often, the "silent member" is dealing with feelings of anxiety about being in the group. There may be a long history of feeling anxious in groups of people -- feeling that they are not safe in a group. They may have past experiences of being criticized or attacked or rejected in group settings. They may also simply be very sensitive to any threats around them and see the potential of danger in a group, and so are responding in a way to keep themselves safe. For some, it may be an act of courage simply to join a group and to show up and sit quietly.

Often, this quiet approach to participation is temporary -- as the person becomes more and more comfortable with the group, they will often speak more and be more engaged in the discussion. The rate at which they get more comfortable varies by the person. For some, being relatively quiet in group settings is a long-standing pattern and is not likely to change a great deal even with time. Because the "silent member" is less disruptive to the group process than the dominating member, your response as leader can be more flexible. Your goal is to ensure they are engaging in the group as much as they can tolerate and that the group can deal with their silence. Again, you might want to think about possible actions in three levels

Initial comments you could make to encourage this person to be engaged in the group include:
- We've heard a lot from a number of people tonight. Mary, I wonder if you have any thoughts you'd like to share.
- How are we doing tonight as far as evenly sharing the discussion? Does everyone feel they are getting a chance to hear from everyone?

The next level of comments might include:
- Mary, I can tell you've got a lot of thoughts about what we are talking about - I wonder if you'd be willing to share?
- We've been talking about wanting everyone in the group to participate. I wonder how other members feel about this. What are your thoughts about those members who tend to more quiet and those who are more talkative?

Advanced comments are often not necessary with the quiet

member, as they are often engaged but less talkative and less disruptive to the group. If the silence is dramatic and persistent, you may want to make comments to them during an individual meeting outside the group. Recognize that comments made during the group that spotlight their silence will make them very anxious, and may drive them out of the group. Comments for an individual meeting outside the group should be supportive and encouraging but seek to elicit more contribution to group discussions. These comments might include:

- Mary, I wanted to check in with you about how you are feeling in the group. You are one of our quieter members, and yet I can tell you are very engaged. I suspect the other group members would love to hear more about your thoughts and experience. Is there something I could do to make it easier for you to share?

THE UNCOMMITTED

The "uncommitted member" tends to have uneven attendance and may talk openly during the group about their mixed feelings about participating in the group. For open groups and groups where attendance and participation is uneven across members, this may not be a problem. For others, the uncommitted member creates a challenge that you may have to deal with.

Sometimes this ambivalence about engaging with the group is caused by conflicting outside commitments. Sometimes it is due more to personality factors that make it difficult for the person to engage in most activities or groups.

The concern for the group, and you as the leader, is that in groups with established memberships and expectations of regular attendance, the uncommitted member becomes a distraction.

For groups where full engagement is important, you may want to consider some of the following comments. Initial comments you might make include:

- Bob, we've been talking about how we feel about coming to the group. Would you be willing to share your thoughts on this?
- As with all groups, different people feel differently about coming and talking with the group. I wonder how people feel about these different levels of commitment.

The next level of comments could include:

- Bob I see that you are back at the meeting tonight. We have missed you. I appreciate your participation when you are here and I would love to see you come more often. Is that a possibility?
- We've been talking about wanting everyone in the group to come and be part of the group. I wonder how other members feel about this. What are your thoughts about those members who are not able to come consistently?

Advanced comments are not necessary if the group is relatively open and can tolerate uneven attendance by a member. If that is not the case, you might want to consider the following:

- Bob, I wanted to check in with you about how you are feeling about being in the group. You are one of our members who is not able to attend as consistently as others, and yet I can tell you are very engaged when you are here. I suspect the other group members love having you as part of the group and would love to see you more. Is there something I could do to make it easier for you to be here more consistently?

THE FIGHTER
Sometimes you have a group member who seems to engage in a

relatively large number of arguments or conflicts with other members or with you as the leader. This may be due to a number of factors. Some people enjoy conflict, finding it stimulating and a way connect to other people. Other people have mixed feelings about connecting with others and use conflict as a way to avoid connection. Still others have very different views from the group and feel it is important to be true to themselves if they are going to be in the group.

As group leader, your concern is that conflict that is either frequent or severe in intensity can damage the connections within the group. Some conflict is normal, but too much is a danger. The "fighter" has a tendency to create frequent conflict which is important to watch and to manage.

Your goal is to help the person and the group to recognize this pattern of engaging in conflict and to talk about it openly if possible. The more it is talked about openly, the more likely the group is to manage the amount and type of conflict that occurs.

Initial comments you might make include:
- We all know that conflict is a normal part of being in any group. Sarah, you've been in several disagreements in the group recently. I wonder if you have thoughts about conflict and how you feel about those conflicts.
- As with all groups, different people feel differently about many things. This sometimes leads to conflict. I wonder how people feel about conflict. How do you typically deal with conflict?

The next level of comments could include:
- Sarah, we've talked in the past about different member's roles in the group. You've been in several conflicts in the group recently. I wonder if this could be a pattern for

you either here or outside the group.
- We've been talking about people's reactions to some of the conflicts in the group recently. I wonder if some of the members see any patterns in the conflict that they'd be willing to share.

Advanced comments may be necessary if the tendency to create conflict continues and is significantly disruptive to the group. Again, consider talking with the person outside of the meeting in a separate place with some privacy. You might want to consider a comment like the following:
- Sarah, I wanted to check in with you about how you are feeling about being in the group. You are one of our members who is very engaged, but who also tends to get into more conflict in the group than others. I'm concerned that that amount of conflict is challenging for the group and is hurting your relationships in the group. You are a valued group member, but I think we need to work toward reducing the amount of conflict. What can we do so that you are not in as much conflict?
- Is this a larger pattern in your life? Could I suggest that you take this into your conversations with your therapist? You might find that will help you get more control over this.

Some examples of less disruptive challenges to watch for:

THE STORY TELLER
The "storyteller" is difficult in that they tend to make comments in the form of stories…. long stories that take up more time than they contribute to the discussion. Unfortunately, the storyteller does not distinguish between parts of a story that are helpful for others to hear, and parts of the story that have little relevance for others. You can sense the quiet tension as the group gets to

know the pattern of responses this member makes. When they start another long story, there is a pregnant silence as members feel frustrated but unsure how to help this person get to the point.

As leader, you are often in the best place to help this person shape their comments in a more helpful frame. You may want to talk with them outside of the group, commenting on your concern that their comments tend to take a long time to make and that briefer comments will likely generate more interaction from the group. You can repeat these comments if the person has trouble changing their behavior. It is good to step in before the frustration of the group members turns into angry comments.

THE FUZZY THINKER

The "fuzzy thinker" often makes comments that are unclear in meaning and leave the group confused. Often there is a silence at the end of the comments because members are not sure what is meant and so not sure how to respond. There are many different styles of thinking, and the "fuzzy thinker" has a particularly unusual style that most others will have difficulty understanding.

As leader, you can often be helpful in trying to clarify what members are saying. You may be doing this often with members who actively contribute but whose thoughts and comments are difficult to understand. There is typically no simple solution to supporting the "fuzzy thinker" beyond patiently helping clarify their comments.

THE CENTER OF DRAMA

Life feels particularly dramatic for some people, and when they join self-help groups, their drama follows them. They may make a lot of comments about the drama in their outside life. They may end up in dramatic conflict or other types of intense interchanges with group members during or outside of the meeting. What is consistent is the intensity and dramatic nature of what happens around them.

In some ways, the "center of drama" brings some positive things to the group, as they can be exciting to hear from and to interact with. Over time, the drama can be emotionally draining for the group, particularly if it keeps the focus on one member. When the drama enters the relationships between group members, it can threaten the trust members are developing and distracting to the focus of the group.

As leader, you will want to watch for members whose comments tend to dominate the group discussion. Keeping the focus fairly evenly distributed will take more work when one or more members tend to be the "center of drama", but that is your task.

When the drama involves group members, you can have your hands full. Helping to referee conflict and reinforce boundaries can help the group survive as this member settles in and learns to trust that the group can care about them and support them even if they don't entertain them with dramatic interactions.

THE OVERWHELMED MEMBER

Any member can present as overwhelmed at some point in the group. Life problems can pile up to a point that we all can feel overwhelmed by the challenge of trying to solve them. When someone comes to a peer support group in an overwhelmed state, it often takes the form of someone who appears very emotional (crying or angry), but it can also look like a member who is unusually quiet and withdrawn. You will be able to see as they are encouraged to speak, that the problems they are facing are so large and/or so many in number, that they are no longer coping well.

At times the group can address this very well, taking time and energy to help the member talk through all that they are facing and then providing encouragement to them as they think about trying to resolve their challenges. At other times, the group will not be able to really help the member and you will have to ask the member to talk after the meeting. Be watchful for signs of a serious crisis and respond in a way that keeps the person safe (see appendix B). Be aware that self-help groups and leaders of those groups are not responsible for solving problems for members, but instead can typically be most helpful by giving them a chance to vent, giving encouragement and empathy, and sharing information about help they may need.

THE "YES, BUT..." MEMBER

The "yes, but..." member shows a predictable pattern of participating in the group by comments about challenges they face, but when others respond with suggestions about how to deal with the challenges, they respond by saying "yes, but....". Any member can say this at times when the group's suggestions are not helpful. When this is such a strong pattern that it seems that the group can never be helpful, you usually are seeing the "yes, but..." member.

In most cases, you are seeing a member who is very ambivalent about getting any help from others, whether it is group members or anyone else in their life. They feel a strong sense of needing help, but they don't want or believe that anyone can actually solve their problem. The group will learn this pattern fairly quickly and will typically stop offering suggestions. This is often the best response, as the person has a long-term lesson to learn -- how to accept help from others. This typically takes some time.

The leader's role is often helping the group cope with the frustration of "yes, but…" responses while the member learns to trust others over time.

THE ADVICE GIVER

The "advice giver" routinely responds to others' comments with advice about how to solve any problem. Occasional advice giving is not a problem, but in general, group members should not be giving each other advice frequently. If you watch how people respond to receiving advice in a group meeting, you will notice that most do not respond well. Instead, many people respond by explaining why that advice will not, or has not worked in the past. They often look tense, as they may feel that the person giving advice is suggesting the problem is relatively easy to solve. They may look puzzled, as they were not looking for advice, but rather to be listened to and supported. They may get very quiet, as they may not want advice and don't want to share if that is going to be the response.

To respond to the member whose comments almost always take the form of advice giving, you may want to remind the group that advice giving tends not to be helpful, and to ask what they personally find to be helpful. You may also want to consider comments such as:

- Bob, instead of giving advice, I wonder if you would be willing to talk about experiences you have had with this type of situation.
- Mary, you just received a lot advice. Was that helpful? What might have been more helpful?
- In general, I think giving advice tends not to be too helpful. Does anyone in the group have thoughts about why we all tend to try to give advice so frequently when we hear about others' problems?

THE SPOKESMAN

The "spokesman" tends to try to talk for others, making comments that sound like they are explaining how other members feel or think about a situation. Like the advice giver, they seem to be trying to help, but their comments typically hurt the group discussion. The spokesman often has not been in the group very long, because most groups will quickly teach members to speak for themselves and not for others. If the group does not, you may want to make a comment like:

- I just want to remind everyone that we've agreed that everyone speaks for themselves. Even if we are trying to help, we should not speak for another group member --- just for ourselves.

THE CARETAKER

The "caretaker" tends to focus on helping other members and does not talk about themselves or their own needs. While this can be helpful for the other group members who need support, the "caretaker" eventually becomes a drain on the group, as they do not share personally and the group doesn't benefit from their full participation.

Like the "yes, but…" member, the "caretaker" is often ambivalent about getting help. They come to meetings for the support, but then only provide support, fearing to make comments that would result in them being supported. Like the "yes, but…" member, time often helps this member to build trust in the group and to start to accept support from others. Some gentle coaxing from you as the group leader can help. Comments like "Jerry, you have been very supportive of others in the group, but I'm less clear on how the group can support you. What can we do to be supportive to you?" can help give them a chance to talk about their own needs. You may have to be patient, as they get comfortable with this type of participation.

CHAPTER 11

DEALING WITH CHALLENGING GROUP SITUATIONS

.

There are situations that arise in peer support groups that predictably feel difficult or at least confusing for the leader. Many represent behaviors by a group that is ambivalent about making progress. The group may sense an opportunity to go deeper in its trust and interactions, but may be afraid to do so. The group may also be stuck and not know how to move forward. Help from a leader who recognizes the situation and knows how to respond may be needed.

THE GROUP IS UNUSUALLY QUIET

Some peer support groups have periods when they are frequently quiet during portions of the meeting. The silence is typically uncomfortable, as if the group doesn't know what to say or as if everyone is afraid to speak. The result is that there is little energy and little movement in the group.

As with every group situation, you'll want to ask "what is this behavior telling me about what the group is experiencing and what the group needs?"

Quiet groups are often feeling stuck before an opportunity to move to a deeper level of involvement. Sometimes this is early in the development of the group and the members just need to learn to trust each other more. Sometimes it is later in the group and the members need to talk about a specific issue or topic that feels challenging and that they are trying to avoid. Topics that groups avoid can be anything, including common issues such as conflict and disagreement, fear of hurting each other's feelings, fear of being different, fear of getting connected, and fear of saying goodbye. In almost every situation, what the group needs is to talk openly about something that they are avoiding.

As a leader, you can help the quiet group in a number of gentle ways, such as making comments:

- You all are very quiet these days. I wonder what all this quiet means about the group?
- You are quiet today. I wonder if the group is uncomfortable talking about something. What might that be?
- The group is fairly quiet tonight. I wonder if it would help for us to check in with each member to see what you are thinking about.

If the quiet continues despite gentle nudges from you, you may want to push a little harder with comments like:

- This is the third meeting in which people don't seem to have much to say. That usually means that people are holding back their thoughts and feelings. What might be so uncomfortable that we can't say it out loud?
- The group is again very quiet this evening. It is starting to feel like we are stuck in some way. Do you have any idea what might be going on that we don't have anything to say to each other?

THE GROUP IS UNUSUALLY NOISY

The noisy group fills much or most of the meeting time with lots of comments and discussion that don't seem to go anywhere. This is not just the occasional meeting when there is lots of unfocused energy or excitement about something. In this difficult situation, there are no comments about members' actual thoughts, feelings or experiences. Instead the opportunity to talk is filled with noisy discussion of things separate from the group members - discussion that feels like a distraction.

The noisy group can be very similar to the quiet group in the underlying dynamic. Instead of being quiet, they often are using noisy discussion to avoid talking about a specific issue or topic that feels challenging.

Like the quiet group, the noisy group will stop avoiding when they actually start to talk about the topics they are avoiding. They may do this naturally over time, but they might need some nudging from you. Some examples of gentle nudges include:

- You are all very talkative these days. I wonder what all the noise is about.

- You all are very busy tonight. I wonder if there is something else that the group may want to talk about that isn't getting said?

If the noisiness continues despite time and gentle nudges, you could push a little harder with comments such as:

- I hear a lot of talking in the group, but I don't hear a lot of members sharing their personal feelings or experiences. I wonder what that is about.

- The group is again very talkative, but sometimes that can be the result of the group avoiding some important topic. Do you have any sense of what we need to be talking about that we are not talking about?

WHEN SOMEONE RELAPSES

For some groups, the issue of members who relapse is a significant concern. There tend to be two different types of concerns, one for groups focusing on substance use or compulsive behaviors in which "relapse" means an episode of returning to the behavior of substance use, gambling etc., and one for groups focused around medical illness in which "relapse" means a deterioration in their physical condition.

For groups that meet around concerns about addiction or compulsive behavior, a member who relapses is a common and important occurrence. The relapse does represent a threat to the wellness and welfare of the group member. At the same time, it tends to threaten the other members' sense of control and safety, often raising anxiety about their own ability to avoid relapse. It is particularly concerning to the group if the person continues to relapse or does not seem concerned about having relapsed.

Common strategies you can use to bring these feelings out into the open include:

- Encourage people to talk about the relapse. In support groups that focus on addiction or compulsive behaviors, relapse should be a regular topic that the group becomes comfortable talking about.

- Encourage the view that in most of these conditions, relapse is predictable and even a "normal" part of recovery for most people. Everyone is at risk.

- Model acceptance and support for the person. Groups can be rejecting toward people who relapse, in part because they feel threatened. Being clear that the people are not a threat -- relapse can happen to anyone -- means accepting and supporting the relapsing member. If you can model acceptance and support, it will help the group be more honest about relapsing.

- Step in when you see the group turning on the person. This can happen quickly, so you want to be active. When someone has relapsed frequently or seems unconcerned about relapsing, the discussion is more difficult, but needs to be done openly and carefully.
- Point out black and white thinking. When groups get anxious, they can resort to simplistic ways of thinking. "No one should be here who relapses", "Relapsing is a terrible failure", "Relapsing means you don't want to recover".
- Bring the group discussion back to how to continue moving toward successful recovery and prevent further relapses.

If the person continues to relapse, help the group intensify its attention and support. If the person doesn't seem to take relapsing seriously, the group will likely need to have more open discussion about how to deal with this truly tricky situation. Again, encourage a message of support for the person, but genuine concern about the behavior. If necessary, individual discussion with the person may be warranted to assess what is going on, and how you can be more helpful.

In rare cases, you may need to encourage the person to get a different type of help - more professional help. Peer support is for those who have a fairly good level of motivation to change.

For groups that meet around concerns about an illness in which relapse means a deterioration in their medical condition, the response will likely be somewhat different. Relapse in a support group for persons with cancer, MS, diabetes or other illnesses that have the risk of relapse, will also raise concerns among group members. Members are typically concerned about the welfare of the member who relapses -- how bad is the relapse? Is there a threat to their life? Will they be able to return to group? Relapses also often trigger anxiety about everyone's welfare, as group members are also at risk for relapse.

Again, open conversation about relapses within this type of group is the key strategy. As leader you want to help ensure open sharing of information that can help the group understand what is happening without violating the privacy or wishes of the person experiencing the relapse. Members may want to know more than the person may want to disclose, and as leader you may need to remind the group of the boundaries on privacy and why those are important to respect. Similarly, you may need to help ensure that members who want to visit a sick group member are doing so in a way that is respectful and helpful. More importantly, you'll want to help the group talk openly about the feelings that the relapse brings up for the group. As talked about before, helping the group to talk through issues openly will eventually lead to more realistic resolution of their fears and concerns than if you let the group avoid talking about a topic that raises their anxiety.

WHEN SOMEONE QUITS ABRUPTLY

The importance of someone leaving a group depends on how involved the person was in the group and how attached the members are to the person. If the person was very involved and/or members were very attached, then the person leaving will have a large impact. If there was little involvement or connection, the person leaving may require limited attention.

In general, it is a good idea for most groups where people get to know each other, that if a person decides to leave the group -- the person leaving should talk about leaving at one or more group meetings. This gives a chance for the person to state that they are leaving and explain why. It also gives a chance for other members to say goodbye and to express their thoughts and feelings about the person's leaving and their involvement in the group. As a leader you will want to mention this expectation occasionally, and encourage anyone planning to leave to come and talk with the group about it at one or more meetings.

Saying goodbye is a natural process that helps bring closure to change in relationships. When there are no goodbyes, the group is left with unresolved questions and feelings. Why did the person leave? Was it something I/we said? Will others leave for the same reason? Even if someone leaves abruptly with no goodbyes, it will be important for most groups to talk about the person leaving, and their thoughts and feelings about why it happened.

WHEN A NUMBER OF NEW MEMBERS JOIN AT ONCE

Most groups can handle one or two new members joining at a time with little trouble, but when a large number of new members join a stable group, it can be a challenge. New members are almost always good to have, but they will need help getting connected. As the leader, you want to assist the group in navigating in this process. Be sure the new members are introduced and get a chance to talk about who they are why they are joining. New members tend to stick together, which is not a bad thing -- they have a lot in common and know that the other new members are typically looking for new connections. Be sure to help older members to interact with the new members. This will help break up any cliques that could be created, and will ease the integration of the new member. If the integration is not going well, you may want to consider pointing this out to the group with the expectation that integrating new members is part of their work. A comment like the following may help.

- I can see that since we have had a lot of new members join recently, we almost have two separate groups going, one with the new members and one with the older members. How can we better build our group so that we are all involved with each other as one group?

SITUATIONS IN WHICH THE GROUP BECOMES DANGEROUS

Every group can be a dangerous at times, which is part of why every group needs at least one leader. Your role includes watching for those moments when the group could enter a discussion that has some potential danger for some or all of the members, and then to step in to nullify the danger. Some examples of potential danger include:

- Group members are angry at a member(s) and are about to attack them. The attack may take the form of intense criticism or hurtful comments, but the goal is to express the anger of the group. While it is good to talk through angry feelings, this situation is dangerous because the angry members are not being careful about how they express their feelings, and are at risk of hurting one or more members while making the group feel unsafe for all.

- Group members feel tense and are at risk for scapegoating a member to bear the brunt of their frustration. Scapegoating is a common behavior in which a group identifies one or more people who get vilified - seen as "all bad". Sometimes this is simply a way to deal with differences between group members, with the most different being scapegoated and alienated. Sometimes it is more complex.

- Sometimes the danger is not from aggressive comments between members, but from efforts to isolate members.

Some groups start to create cliques and to create "in-groups" and "out-groups". Those in the in-group feel more connected to the group as a whole, while those in the out-group(s) feel isolated and unaccepted. Often this is evidence that the group is not talking openly about the differences between all members, not talking about the tension between being connected with others while recognizing that we are all different.

These are just a few examples of how groups can be dangerous to its members. Again, as leader, you hopefully can help identify when the group is starting down the road to acting out in a way that can be dangerous. Red flags to look for include (1) mounting tension and conflict, (2) when negative feelings start to focus on one or two members, (3) when the group starts to divide into subgroups that are tense with each other.

Once you see danger approaching, you have a number of strategies you can use to help the group work through the danger in a constructive way. In each situation, it is important to recognize that there is something important for the group to learn. In order to learn the underlying lesson, the group needs to talk about what is going on in the group in a way that avoids taking any destructive action. To help the group do this you might want to try some of the following.

Help slow down the discussion long enough to invite members to start to talk openly about what they are feeling. You will have to be active, even assertive in these situations. For example, comments like the following might help:

- I wonder if we can slow this conversation down a bit. I'd like everyone to step back and comment on what you are feeling.
- I'm afraid I'm confused about what we are really talking

about. Seems like there is a lot more going on in our conversation than is reflected in the words we are saying. Let's step back a moment and talk about what we each are feeling.

Stop the destructive action and divert the energy toward reflecting on the group's behavior. This can be done with comments like the following:

- I want to remind the group that our comfort agreement says that we don't make hurtful or cutting comments to each other. This conversation is going in that direction. I'd like everyone to stop and take a deep breath. There is some reason this is coming up and we want to backtrack until we can figure what it is.

- I need to stop the discussion at this point, as people are in danger of saying hurtful things -- that is not what this group is about. This usually occurs when we are not talking honestly about other feelings. Can we back away from this topic and start to think for a minute about what we might be avoiding?

Challenge the group to take a very different direction toward understanding what they are doing.

- I would like to observe that the group seems to be dividing more and more into subgroups. Can we take 10 minutes to talk about what this is about. Why are these divisions taking place and what do they say about how we all are feeling?

- The group seems very tense tonight, bordering on angry. Can we back up and look at what feelings we are avoiding that we feel a need to be so tense with each other? I think there is something more to this than meets the eye.

THE DISAPPEARING GROUP

Just as most people love to join a lively group, they hate to be in a group in which others are leaving. There is a deep fear of being the last person left as group members leave - regardless of the reason.

When you see a series of members leaving, you can rest assured that the group experiences this as a threatening situation. There will be anxiety about members leaving that can lead to more members leaving.

Your job as leader is to act quickly to help identify why people are leaving before the remaining members feel that the group is not safe to continue with. You will want to talk to those who have left (if they are willing to share openly about why they left) and with those who are still in the group, looking for experiences or concerns that might make others leave. By moving quickly to collect information, and then feeding that information back to the group to discuss openly, you give the group an opportunity to address whatever underlying problems are there. At times there are no problems to address, just some members who had to leave for personal reasons. In that case, the group gets to see that and adapt to it.

THE PASSIVE GROUP

Groups, like individuals, can be slow to take action when it is called for. The passive group tends to respond slowly when opportunities to move forward come up. You may experience it as feeling that the group has little direction or energy. It may seem that the group is waiting for someone or something to happen. There may be silences that suggest no one knows what to do.

Any group can find itself in a place where it takes a passive stance towards moving forward. Often this reflects a sense of anxiety about taking that next step. The anxiety may be fear of failure or criticism. It may also be fear of taking the next step successfully - fear of what will come with success. Often, if someone in the group can simply help members talk openly about the situation, the group will move to a more active stance

When a group has a stable pattern of taking a passive stance, you as the leader have a more difficult challenge. This may reflect the fact that many people in the group tend to take a passive stance toward life or toward their problems. It may also reflect the fact that the group feels a lot of anxiety about being a group - anxiety about connecting with each other and talking openly. As leader, your task is to try to understand what is behind the passivity, and help the group recognize the need to take a more active stance. Helping them voice their anxieties often leads them to start moving forward.

CHAPTER 12

VARIOUS FORMATS FOR GROUPS

There are a variety of formats that groups can take, each
variation having advantages and disadvantages. If you are
developing a new group, you will want to match the format to
the situation you are trying to address. If you are working with
an existing group, you will want to recognize the advantages and
disadvantages of the existing format, and find ways to maximize
the advantages while minimizing the disadvantages.

DROP-IN VS. MEMBERSHIP GROUPS

Drop-in groups are open to anyone who knows about the group
and wants to attend a meeting. This is the format with the least
restriction on who attends the meeting. The advantages of this
format include the following:

- There is no barrier to attendance for anyone - no prior
  tasks or steps prospective members have to take before
  coming to a meeting, providing very easy access.
- There is no commitment to a certain level of attendance
  or participation, again, minimizing the barriers to access
  for potential participants who are not able to commit to
  a minimum level of participation.

The disadvantages of this format include the following:

- The lack of any minimal requirements for attendance can result in people attending who are not appropriate for the group, who do not know the basics of participation. This can result in some confusion if people attend who are not able to participate or should not participate.

- A drop-in group provides the least warning to the group and to you as leader, as to who is coming to each meeting. There may be many or few attendees. There may be many people who the group does not know, and who may not come back. That level of uncertainty can make it more difficult for some attendees to form a strong sense of who is in the group, and thus can slow down their attachment to the group as a whole. It also means that you as leader will have to be even more ready for the unexpected, as you'll never know who may come to a meeting.

- The lack of a minimal commitment for participation often results in more uneven participation by some members, and thus the group is slower to form a strong sense of identity and trust. When most attendees do not attend on a predictable basis, the group can be very slow to develop any sense of cohesion.

In a "membership" group, there is an expectation that anyone attending a meeting has met with you as the leader to find out about the group, what the mission of the group is and what the requirements of participation are. It is also expected that they have made some type of commitment for participation, whatever the expectation is for members. The advantages of this format include:

- Attendees have been screened and oriented to the group and so are more likely to feel that the mission and format of the group fit their needs. This results in less turnover in attendance and less chance that people will come who are not appropriate for the group. This can result in less uncertainty in the meetings for you as the leader and for the other members.

- Attendance tends to be more steady, as people who are not appropriate for the group, and those who cannot make a minimal commitment to participate do not attend. Continuity in participants helps the group build trust and cohesion more quickly, which can allow the group to talk at a deeper level of experience.

The disadvantage of the "membership" group is that the screening process can limit access to people who could benefit from the group but are not willing to make the minimum commitment.

WIDE- VS. NARROWLY-FOCUSED GROUPS

There can be a great deal of variation in the degree of focus of peer support groups. For example, there are groups for victims of trauma, for victims of specific types of trauma (military trauma vs. assault vs. rape vs. motor vehicle accident), and even for certain types of victims of certain types of trauma (e.g. women over the age of 50 who are victims of rape). Groups with a relatively wide focus have a number of advantages including:

- They have more potential members, and so it can be easier to recruit new members.
- The variation in experiences of the members can lead to broader discussions that help the group see larger themes across the experiences of members.

Some of the disadvantages include:

- The wider focus can feel too broad to some potential participants, and so they may be less interested in joining.

- The variation in experiences can make it harder for people to talk about shared aspects of the experience. This can slow the group's ability to build a sense of mutual understanding and trust, and thus the group may take more time to get to the same level of discussion than a group with a more narrow focus.

In contrast, groups with a more narrow focus have a number of valuable advantages including:

- The narrow focus makes it easier for prospective members to see that the group fits their experience, which can make it easier to recruit new members and easier for members to quickly feel connected to the group. Homogeneous groups tend to grow more quickly, and a narrow focus for a group adds to the homogeneity.
- The narrow focus can help the group, and you as the leader, to focus on more specific topics quickly. This can allow the discussion to move to a deeper level more quickly.

The disadvantages of a narrow focus include:

- The narrow focus limits the number of people who will be able to join the group, and so may create a greater challenge for recruitment and replacement of members.
- The narrow focus can emphasize the sense that the group has a special shared experience or status that others do not have, resulting in lost opportunities to see broader commonalities with other people and other experiences.

TIME LIMITED VS. UNLIMITED

While most peer support groups are not time limited, some are. For example, you may want to set up a new group that will meet for 12 weeks to study a certain book together, or a group that will meet for 6 months to help a group of people who are going through a transition at work. Time limits have some advantages that you may want to consider, including:

- The limited time commitment will encourage some people to participate, as they will feel that they can commit to something of limited duration.

- The time commitment can create a sense of urgency that pushes the group to work more quickly. This can motivate members to be more active in their participation, resulting in more lively discussions, more risk-taking and a greater effort by members to apply the conclusions of the discussion to their outside lives.

In contrast, the disadvantages include the following:

- The time limitation will discourage potential participants who are looking for on-going support from a group.

- The natural processes of developing trust and connection in a group take time. If the time frame for the group is too short, some of the most desirable aspects of peer support groups will not be able to fully develop.

GROUPS WITH PROFESSIONAL STAFF ATTENDING

By definition, peer support groups are made up of laypeople supporting each other. If a professional provider leads the group, the group is no longer a true peer support/self-help group. It is important to note that terminology can be used differently, and there a large number of "support groups" that are led by professional clinicians, particularly in clinical settings.

There has been some experimenting with including clinical providers in peer support groups in a way that does not violate the definition of peer support. For example, some groups have included a professional staff in the initial meetings of a new group to help the group get established and to encourage confidence in people considering whether they should join the group. The initial meetings of any new group can be some of the most challenging, and so having an experienced provider in attendance as a consultant can be a valuable resource, particularly for relatively new leaders. It also encourages confidence in people who may be anxious about committing to a peer support group due to concerns about whether the group will be safe and effective

Other groups have included clinical providers as regular members -- not as a leader, but as a support or on-going consultant to the leader. Again, this can be helpful for what an experienced provider can bring in terms of support to the leaders and to the group members, and the confidence they can help establish. The disadvantage is that some potential members may be less willing to join a group, or may be less open with their comments in a group, if a professional is attending.

It is important that any professional who does attend be very committed to the definition of the group as "peer support" and so avoid creating a group therapy model, or a group in which they play a role as an active expert who dominates the discussion.

Possibly the most effective use of professional staff in peer support groups is the occasional inclusion of providers as consultants to the group <u>by invitation</u> to address a specific question or issue. Groups will find that some topics or challenges can be better understood with the input of a provider. Inviting a provider to answer questions can enrich the discussion without changing the nature of the group.

GROUPS WITH FAMILY MEMBERS AND FRIENDS ATTENDING

Many groups are open to, and encourage attendance by family and friends of group members. Some groups limit this to family and friends of members of the group, and others are less restrictive. The advantages of including family and friends include:

- Family and friends often have a unique and valuable perspective on the common issue, and so can make comments that provide useful insight to other members.

- For groups focused around clinical and/or life problems, family and friends often share the burden of managing those problems, and so including them in the discussion provides support to them while emphasizing the fact that they are part of the solution.

Disadvantages of including family and friends include:

- Some members may not feel as comfortable talking in front of family and friends, and so the group may be slower to build trust and connection, and the discussion may develop more slowly. This seems to be dependent on the focus of the group and the preferences of the members.

- Often, the needs of family members and friends are different from the needs of the central members. Including them can result in the focus of discussion being split between the needs of the central members and the family/friends. This can be less satisfying to all. It is for this reason that some organizations like AA, have established separate meetings and organizations for family and friends (e.g. Al-Anon, Alateen).

LARGE GROUPS (>15 MEMBERS)

There is a traditional view that effective groups should have somewhere between 6 and 15 members. While there are advantages to this traditional size, I have seen very successful groups of more than fifty attendees and with four or fewer members. As a leader, you will want to think though the advantages of working with a large or small group.

The key advantages of a large group include:

- Large groups often result because the group is open and active and so people are very engaged and actively recruiting others. Limiting the size of the group can limit the vitality of a group.

- Large groups have more perspectives and more variety in membership, which can add to the discussion.

- Large groups can provide more opportunity for members to sit quietly and listen to others. For members who are new to care, are ambivalent about care, or who are anxious about participating, the potential of sitting quietly and learning from the group without pressure to speak can be very attractive. Often, as they listen to others, they will grow in confidence and will become more active. Without the opportunity to sit quietly and speak when they are more comfortable, some potential members will not join.

Some of the disadvantages of a large group include:

- By necessity, the inclusion of more members results in less individual time and attention for the average member. Some potential members are looking for a place where they can talk and so large groups look less attractive to them.

- Large groups can be more challenging to manage for you as the leader, as they often have more active agendas among the members, and sometimes have a greater number of members who require special attention and support.

SMALL GROUPS (<6 MEMBERS)

Groups with five or fewer members are not uncommon and can be very successful, but it is worth considering the costs and benefits of this format. The advantages of a small group include:

- There is more time per participant, and so the group tends to build trust more quickly, and so can move more deeply into topics at a quicker pace.
- The depth of the relationships can develop more quickly and so you may find more support occurring outside of the meeting, and more connection between members.
- Smaller groups can be easier to support, so they may be less work for you.

Some of the key disadvantages of small groups include:

- Small groups have fewer perspectives and so the discussion can be more limited and less helpful.
- If the group is too small, some members will feel there is too much attention on them -- too much pressure to talk. This can discourage some from joining.
- If the group is very small (2 or 3 members), prospective members may wonder why there are not more members, and so building the group can be more difficult.

IN-PROGRAM VS. COMMUNITY-BASED GROUPS

Some peer support groups occur on the site of clinical, social service, or court-based programs. Sometimes this reflects the fact that the program is sponsoring the group or even staffing it with Peer Specialists. Sometimes this simply reflects the fact that programs want to have self-help groups holding meetings on their site, either to encourage their patients/clients to attend, or as a service to the community.

Recently, there has been growing interest by clinical programs in helping patients/clients become more active in community-based activities, including peer support groups based in the community. This reflects the growing realization that community integration is an important overall goal of care which requires the involvement of patients in community-based activities. Given these emerging trends, it is important for you to recognize the impact of developing a new group in a clinical vs. community setting.

The advantages of a peer support group that occurs within a clinical program or is co-located with a clinical program include:

- The clinical program can be a more active partner in referring people to the group.
- There is better integration of what people are working on in the clinical setting and in the support group. This can create more shared experience among members, as many or most will have participated in treatment in the same setting.
- Communication with clinical providers can be easier, and so when appropriate, can lead to better care.
- Clinical programs can often provide better space than community sites.

The disadvantages that should be considered include:

- The clinical program may tend to influence, or try to influence the group more than the group may want.

- There may be a temptation to be sloppy around the use of signed releases of information for communication about participants between the peer support group leaders and clinicians. This is easily addressed by being conscientious around legal boundaries.

- Sometimes, peer support groups that take place in clinical settings can start to act like therapy groups. This is an important danger, as you don't want the peer group to lose the qualities of a self-help focus. As a facilitator, you don't want to be in a group that is doing group therapy, as that is outside your responsibilities and could lead to situations that you will have trouble managing. This would also raise concerns among your clinical partners.

- If one of the clinical needs of group members is to get more established in the community, and more connected to the community, then holding the group in a clinical setting can send the wrong message -- that support takes place in clinical settings and not in the community.

The advantages of groups that are located in the community include:

- The group can be more accessible to potential members in that community. This can lead to better social integration into that community, as members make connections and those relationships lead to activities together outside the group.

- Holding a group in the community gives a clear message that social support exists in the community and recovery needs to be in the community. This likely encourages better community integration outcomes.

- Community-based groups can be more independent, as there is little temptation to rely on a clinical program.

Disadvantages of community-based groups include:

- The opportunities to set up active referral processes from clinical programs to the group will take more work on your part, and so the flow of new participants may be slower.

- The clinical supports that are occasionally needed are not as convenient, and so you as leader will have to set up connections to help you when participants need referrals and urgent supports.

PHONE AND WEB-BASED PEER SUPPORT GROUPS

The use of technology to create peer support groups with easy access to virtually anyone is rapidly expanding. These are true support groups, with members interacting with each other during a set period of time, as opposed to listservs, and other web-based tools in which people communicate but not as a group and not in real time.

Phone and web-based peer support groups are an important development that is likely to further accelerate the growth in the number and scope of support groups functioning around the world. They allow people in countries and regions with few face-to-face support groups, to join a group. They are also important for groups that focus on experiences and conditions that are so rare that they affect only a few people even in large communities.

A growing body of research has been focusing on the value of phone or web-based support groups (See appendix A). The majority of the evidence suggests that these support groups serve the same purpose as face-to-face groups, and are beneficial in the same ways for participants.

CHAPTER 13

THE RANGE OF APPLICATIONS

The use of organized peer support groups is common and has been rapidly expanding over the past 50 years, both in the number of people participating in groups, in the geographical area in which groups are available, and in the range of healthcare and life situations for which specialized peer support groups are available. To gain some sense of the scope of groups available, this chapter provides a brief review of some of the most common types of groups you are likely to find available near you.

You will see below that there is a wide range of models of support that can help inform how you think about any group you may lead. It is also helpful to know that there are many groups available, as you are likely to find group members who will need referrals to other types of peer support groups. There are also times when you may want to consult with, or develop relationships with other peer support group leaders. Hopefully you will see from the following, that there are many groups in almost every geographic area, and so there are plenty of opportunities to connect with other group leaders.

To help think about the variety of groups, I have tried to organize them around broad categories of focus. I have highlighted those supported or at least cataloged by a national or international organization, and links to directories for self-help groups supported by these organizations can be found in Chapter 15. This is not to downplay the number and importance of self-help groups that are not aligned with large organizations. There are many groups that are aligned only with local organizations and others that are not aligned with any organization. They play an important role in providing support in many areas, and you'll want to make connections with those groups and group leaders as well.

GROUPS RELATED TO THE MISUSE OF DRUGS AND ALCOHOL

Peer support groups have been such a key element of recovery from misuse of drugs and alcohol that when people hear the term "self-help group", they often think of AA. The reality is that there are more self-help groups for substance-related conditions than any other type of group, and those groups are available to a larger portion of the world than any other. This may contribute to that fact that, more than any other application, there is a substantial body of research evaluating the impact of peer support groups for people struggling with drug and alcohol use disorders. While researchers are not in full agreement as to all of the benefits of participating in a peer support group, there is good agreement on the basic benefits and dynamics of self-help group. Appendix A summarizes some of the key findings.

Alcoholics Anonymous (AA) is by far, the largest organization supporting peer support groups focusing on a clinical problem. AA defines itself as a "mutual aid fellowship" to help alcoholics "stay sober and help other alcoholics achieve sobriety". Founded by Bill Wilson and Dr. Bob Smith in 1935, AA relies on the "Twelve Steps" as the core of the curriculum or program philosophy. There is also a key book written by the founders and other early members, often referred to as "the Big Book"

(Alcoholics Anonymous: The Story of How More Than One Hundred Men Have Recovered from Alcoholism) which provides content that many members use as part of their work in AA. AA participation involves a spiritual element, reflecting the fact that the organization has its roots in the <u>Oxford Group</u>, a non-denominational Christian religious movement originating in the early 1900's that was associated with Oxford University.

AA has an extensive network of peer support meetings, as many as 100,000 located in a wide range of locations around the world. There are millions of members, though attendance at many meetings is open and so there is no easy way to identify the true number of members. Because of its relatively long history, AA has worked out a wide variety of organizational issues that are valuable for self-help organizations, and so has become a model for many developing organizations.

Each AA group is seen as a self-governing unit, with the larger organization primarily playing an advisory role. Members are expected to remain anonymous in public media, with the expectation that groups focus solely on providing peer support and avoid getting draw into other agendas. There are a number of informal activities that are voluntary in nature (organizing the meetings, collecting funds for coffee, serving as "sponsors" for other members, etc.).

AA meetings fall into a number of common formats. "Open meetings" can be attended by anyone while "closed meetings" are limited to those in recovery from alcohol dependence. There are also "speaker" meetings which focus on the stories of a few speakers, "discussion" meetings which involve a more wide ranging conversation, and meetings focused around the study of a specific book. While some meetings are identified with specific target groups (e.g. men, women, newcomers, LGBTQ groups, etc.) the basic format of meetings is the same regardless of location. AA promotes an abstinence model of recovery, with progress in recovery marked by "chips" to document length of successful abstinence. AA also supports individual mentoring relationships outside of meetings, by encouraging members with significant successful sobriety to serve as "sponsors" for other members.

Meetings tend to vary widely in focus, size and quality. There are formal methods to find meetings, including web-based guides and written listings. There is also a great deal of informal discussion between attendees about meetings that are available and the strengths and weaknesses of specific meetings (see Chapter 15 for connections to AA resources).

As originally stated by AA, the *Twelve Steps* are:

1. *We admitted we were powerless over alcohol - that our lives had become unmanageable.*

2. *Came to believe that a power greater than ourselves could restore us to sanity.*

3. *Made a decision to turn our will and our lives over to the care of God as we understood Him.*

4. *Made a searching and fearless moral inventory of ourselves.*

5. *Admitted to God, to ourselves, and to another human being the exact nature of our wrongs.*

6. *Were entirely ready to have God remove all these defects of character.*

7. *Humbly asked Him to remove our shortcomings.*

8. *Made a list of all persons we had harmed, and became willing to make amends to them all.*

9. *Made direct amends to such people wherever possible, except when to do so would injure them or others.*

10. *Continued to take personal inventory, and when we were wrong, promptly admitted it.*

11. *Sought through prayer and meditation to improve our conscious contact with God as we understood Him, praying only for knowledge of His will for us and the power to carry that out.*

12. *Having had a spiritual awakening as the result of these steps, we tried to carry this message to alcoholics, and to practice these principles in all our affairs.*

For family and friends affected by someone's drinking, related peer support group organizations have developed (Al-Anon for family and friends, Alateen for teenage family and friends).

AA has spawned a range of related peer support organizations that focus on other substance use disorders or troubling behaviors, and that often share some elements of format and organization.

Al-Anon and Alateen are elements of an international network of support groups for family and friends of people with an alcohol problem. Al-Anon is a broader group, while Alateen is designed for teenagers, with the idea that each group has a need for different types of support. Like AA, Al-Anon and Alateen meetings have variation in format, with some meetings being open to non-members, some meetings having a focus on the 12-steps or another discussion topic, etc. The network of groups is fairly extensive and well-organized.

Cocaine Anonymous (CA): Modeled after AA, CA provides a network of peer support groups for adults seeking recovery from cocaine use (including "crack" cocaine), as well as other "mind altering substances". CA uses the 12-step format along with other elements of AA. It was founded in Los Angeles in 1982 and has spread across North America and Europe.

Crystal Meth Anonymous (CMA): Similar to CA, CMA is an AA spinoff that uses the 12-step peer support format to help those with problems related to abuse of crystal methamphetamine ("crystal meth") to establish and sustain abstinence. Like CA, they state that many CMA members find it more helpful to meet with other adults who are seeking recovery from crystal meth use, as opposed to a broader group dealing with different substance use problems. Founded in 1994, CMA may be one of the smaller AA spinoffs, but it appears to be growing in number and in the range of areas in which it is available.

Dual Recovery Anonymous describes itself as a "Fellowship of men & women who meet to support each other in our common recovery from an emotional or psychiatric illness and chemical dependency". They use a 12-step model to help people address the challenge of both a substance use and a mental health disorder.

Families Anonymous if a 12-step groups for family and friends of someone with a substance use problem. Unlike Al-Anon, Nar-Anon and Coc-Anon, Families Anonymous is not substance-specific. Families Anonymous also seeks to focus explicitly on issues of co-dependency.

Life Ring Secular Recovery (LRSR) is another non-profit network of self-help groups seeking to support adults who want to achieve abstinence from alcohol or drugs. Unlike AA, LRSR does not focus on spirituality as a key part of recovery, though religion is not discouraged. LRSR emphasizes a wider range of methods to achieving abstinence, stating that each person must find an "individual path" to abstinence, but by doing so together, members can support each other's efforts. LRSR operates in many large US cities, and in some sites in Canada and Europe.

Marijuana Anonymous (MA) is another 12-step organization that focuses on abuse of a single substance. MA is active mostly in large cities in the US and Canada, with some meetings internationally. There are in-person, phone, and online meetings, as well as meetings for family members.

Moderation Management (MM) provides a network of self-help groups that seek to help the "problem drinker" in contrast to the alcoholic. In contrast to AA, MM uses a harm reduction model to help problem drinkers reduce and manage their alcohol use in an effort to reduce the damage of problem drinking and avoid progress to addiction. There is some evidence that MM often serves as a stepping stone to abstinence and to participation in a broader group of self-help organizations.

MM uses a core statement called the "Nine Steps Toward Moderation and Toward Lifestyle Changes":

1. *Attend meetings or on-line groups and learn about the program of Moderation Management.*

2. *Abstain from alcoholic beverages for 30 days and complete steps three through six during this time.*

3. *Examine how drinking has affected your life.*

4. *Write down your life priorities.*

5. *Take a look at how much, how often, and under what circumstances you had been drinking.*

6. *Learn the MM guidelines and limits for moderate drinking.*

7. *Set moderate drinking limits and start weekly "small steps" toward balance and moderation in other areas of your life.*

8. Review your progress and update your goals.

9. Continue to make positive lifestyle changes and attend meetings whenever you need ongoing support or would like to help newcomers.

MM groups operate in many US and Canadian cities, as well as in Europe.

Narcotics Anonymous (NA) is the largest spinoff from AA, and the largest peer support organization for adults struggling with substance use disorders (SUD) other than alcohol. It was founded in 1953 and is now global in scope. While AA is limited to those struggling with recovery from alcohol problems, NA is open to those in recovery from any substance use disorder.

The format and content of NA is similar to that found in AA, with a focus on abstinence as the primary path to recovery and the use of the 12-steps as a means of establishing and developing recovery. Like AA, a key part of participation is choosing a sponsor, who is someone who has time and experience in recovery and who can provide support outside of NA meetings.

Nar-Anon is complementary to Al-Anon, serving as a 12-step program for family and friends of people with a drug addiction. Nar-Anon has a smaller network of groups than Al-Anon, but the list is growing.

Nicotine Anonymous uses a 12-step model to help members quit using nicotine products. As in most peer support groups focusing on substance use, participants can be using other formal treatment options as well. Groups exist in the US and in some parts of the world, though the number of groups is not large.

Secular Organization for Sobriety (SOS) is non-profit network of autonomous self-help groups that use a non-spiritual model of recovery to help attendees achieve abstinence. It supports a broader network of meetings than LSRS, with meetings in the US, Canada and around the world.

Self-Management and Recovery Training Recovery (SMART Recovery) is a non-profit organization that supports a network of groups for people seeking abstinence from alcohol or drugs through "self-empowerment and self-directed change". SMART Recovery groups use a cognitive-behavioral model to teach specific tools and techniques within a 4-point program:

1. *Enhancing and maintaining motivation to abstain.*

2. *Coping with urges.*

3. *Problem solving (managing thoughts, feelings, and behaviors).*

4. *Lifestyle balance (balancing momentary and enduring satisfactions).*

SMART Recovery groups operate across the US and Canada as well as in Europe.

Women for Sobriety (WFS) is a non-profit that focuses on helping women achieve sobriety from alcohol and other substance use. The program states that its focus on women is a response to early research data suggesting that AA may be more effective for men than woman. WFS uses an abstinence-based model that has a greater emphasis on psychological growth, reflected in their "Thirteen Statements of Positivity".

1. *I have a life-threatening problem that once had me.*
   I now take charge of my life and my disease. I accept the responsibility.

2. *Negative thoughts destroy only myself.*
   My first conscious sober act must be to remove negativity from my life.

3. *Happiness is a habit I will develop.*
   Happiness is created, not waited for.

4. *Problems bother me only to the degree I permit them to.*
    I now better understand my problems and do not permit problems to overwhelm me.

5. *I am what I think.*
    I am a capable, competent, caring, compassionate woman.

6. *Life can be ordinary or it can be great.*
    Greatness is mine by a conscious effort.

7. *Love can change the course of my world.*
    Caring becomes all important.

8. *The fundamental object of life is emotional and spiritual growth.*
    Daily I put my life into a proper order, knowing which are the priorities.

9. *The past is gone forever.*
    No longer will I be victimized by the past. I am a new person.

10. *All love given returns.*
    I will learn to know that others love me.

11. *Enthusiasm is my daily exercise.*
    I treasure all moments of my new life.

12. *I am a competent woman and have much to give life.*
    This is what I am and I shall know it always.

13. *I am responsible for myself and for my actions.*
    I am in charge of my mind, my thoughts, and my life.

GROUPS RELATED TO BROADER MENTAL HEALTH CONDITIONS (E.G. DEPRESSION, ANXIETY, BIPOLAR DISORDER, SCHIZOPHRENIA)

There is a large and growing array of peer support groups for adults dealing with mental health conditions other than substance use disorders. Some are organized around a specific disorder or combination of disorders, while others are organized around the theme of recovery or some aspect of recovery. Many are independent of any national organization, and some are supported by clinical providers. Here are a few of those with national and/or international networks.

The Anxiety and Depression Association of America (ADAA) provides a range of peer support groups focused on anxiety and depression, with some specialized groups for more specific problems like agoraphobia and PTSD. The groups are active in the United States and Canada.

The Depression Bipolar Support Alliance (DBSA) offers a network of peer support groups for adults with depression and/or bipolar disorder. DBSA states they support over 700 support groups around the US, and has a growing network of on-line support groups as well.

Depressed Anonymous (DA) is 12-step program designed for adults struggling with depression, and their family members. It is a relatively small 12-step program, holding meetings in just a portion of the United States, but appears to be growing.

Dialectical Behavior Therapy (DBT) Peer Support Groups are not organized under one organization, but supported by a range of organizations. DBT was developed primarily for adults diagnosed with Borderline Personality Disorder, but many adults have found the skills taught through DBT to be helpful. DBT peer support groups meet for mutual support and to continue skill development related to this model of care.

<u>Dual Recovery Anonymous</u> (described previously under 'groups related to misuse of drugs and alcohol') refers to itself as a "Fellowship of men & women who meet to support each other in our common recovery from an emotional or psychiatric illness and chemical dependency". They use a 12-step model to help people address the challenge of both a substance use and a mental health disorder.

<u>Emotions Anonymous (EA)</u> is a peer support network modeled after AA, but with a very broad focus of serving adults seeking recovery from "emotional difficulties", including "depression, anger, broken or strained relationships, grief, anxiety, low self-esteem, panic, abnormal fears, resentment, jealousy, guilt, despair, fatigue, tension, boredom, loneliness, withdrawal, obsessive and negative thinking, worry, compulsive behavior" and other emotional issues.

<u>The International Obsessive Compulsive Foundation</u> provides a directory for a diverse group of peer support groups around the United States focused on those suffering with Obsessive Compulsive Disorder (OCD) and related disorders, as well as for their family and friends. Most groups focus on OCD, but some focus on targeted subgroups of people such as those with Body Dysmorphic Disorder or those with "Perfectionism".

<u>National Alliance on Mental Illness (NAMI)</u> sponsors and supports two networks of peer support groups across the United States, one for adults in recovery from a mental illness (NAMI Connection Recovery Support Groups) and one for family members of someone with a mental illness (NAMI Family Support Groups). NAMI is a grass-roots organization that has grown in size and influence in the past decade, and has been very active in expanding peer support offerings around the United States.

Postpartum Progress is a non-profit organization that supports peer-to-peer support, including support for a network of peer support groups across the United States for women with postpartum depression. Postpartum Support International also coordinates a network of support groups for mothers struggling with postpartum depression, and other family members.

PTSD - The Gift from Within: Family Members and Caregivers for Adults with PTSD, provides a small but growing listing of support groups relevant to PTSD in the US and internationally. This network is diverse in the format for the groups and does not have a single model to provide of support.

Recovery International / The Abraham Low Institute (RI/TALI) Recovery International offers meetings for adults with mental health issues seeking to lead more "peaceful and productive lives".   Groups include peer support and training on self - management skills developed by Dr. Abraham Low to help people change behavior and attitudes, mostly based on cognitive-behavioral principals.

Schizophrenics Anonymous (SA) is a peer support group network that was started in 1985 and has grown to include support groups in the United States and eight other countries. Modeled after AA, SA has adapted a number of the key AA elements, including a revised set of 6 steps:

- *I SURRENDER... I admit I need help. I can't do it alone.*

- *I CHOOSE... I choose to be well. I take full responsibility for my choices and realize the choices I make directly influence the quality of my days.*

- *I BELIEVE... I now come to believe that I have been provided with great inner resources and I will use these resources to help myself and others.*

- *I FORGIVE… I forgive myself for all the mistakes I have made. I also forgive and release everyone who has injured or harmed me in any way.*

- *I UNDERSTAND… I now understand that erroneous, self-defeating thinking contributes to my problems, failures, unhappiness and fears. I am ready to have my belief system altered so my life can be transformed.*

- *I DECIDE… I make a decision to turn my life over to the care of a higher power/God, AS I UNDERSTAND that higher power/God, surrendering my will and false beliefs. I ask to be changed in depth.*

<u>Wellness Recovery Action Plan (WRAP) Support Groups</u> are peer support groups set up in a range of settings using the WRAP materials developed by Maryellen Copeland (2015) as core content for a peer support group focused on promoting wellness and recovery in adults with mental illness.

GROUPS RELATED TO TROUBLING BEHAVIORS (E.G. DISORDERED EATING, GAMBLING OR SEX)

There are a number of peer support organizations focusing on troubling behaviors that some would call compulsive or addictive behaviors. While some may qualify as a mental illness, I have put these groups in this separate section because of their similarities.

GROUPS FOCUSING ON BEHAVIOR AROUND EATING
<u>Anorexics and Bulimics Anonymous (ABA)</u> is a non-profit 12-step organization that supports an international network of peer support groups for adults with anorexia or bulimia.

<u>Eating Disorders Anonymous</u>, is another non-profit organization that uses a 12-step model of peer support to help members

recover from an eating disorder. They support groups around the United States and in several European countries.

The National Eating Disorders Association provides a directory of peer support groups that focus on eating disorders and related topics in North America, the South Pacific and in the US Armed Forces.

Overeaters Anonymous (OA) calls itself a " fellowship of individuals who, through shared experience, strength, and hope, are recovering from compulsive overeating." Using a 12-step approach, this peer support network serves adults in over 80 countries. There are open and closed meetings, as well as special focus, special population meetings, and virtual meetings.

GROUPS FOCUSING ON BEHAVIOR AROUND MONEY
Debtors Anonymous (DA) uses an AA format to help adults deal with compulsive borrowing, often a part of compulsive shopping or spending beyond their means. DA has three stated goals: to help members stop incurring unsecured (no collateral) debt, to share openly with others, and to reach out to those who need help. There is a subgroup of meetings designed for those who are self-employed called Business Debtors Anonymous.

Gamblers Anonymous (GA) uses a 12-step approach to help adults with problem gambling. Begun in 1957, GA has spread across the United States and to over 50 countries. To help people determine if they have a gambling problem, GA offers the "Twenty Questions". For family and friends affected by problem gambling, there is an affiliated network of groups called Gam-Anon. Bettors Anonymous is a very similar organization with a smaller network of support groups.

GROUPS FOCUSING ON SEXUAL BEHAVIOR

Sex Addicts Anonymous (SAA) is one of at least five separate organizations that use an AA format to provide peer support for adults seeking recovery from compulsive or addictive sexual behavior. Members are encouraged to define their own target goal of 'sexual sobriety', and to pursue that goal while they respect others who may have the same or different goals.

Sexual Compulsives Anonymous (SCA) is similar to SAA in focus, but has some key differences. SCA states that their mission is to help members "to stay sexually sober and to help others to achieve sexual sobriety", though they do not define sexual sobriety as abstinence. Members are encouraged to define sexual sobriety for themselves and to use this goal as the target in developing a written "sexual recovery plan". SCA developed in 80's or 90's, originally serving primarily gay and bisexual men, though it has broadened the type of participants in recent years.

Sex and Love Addicts Anonymous (SLAA), sometimes referred to the "Augustine Fellowship", is another 12-step program that focuses on helping adults struggling with compulsive sexual behavior. Founded in 1976, SLAA has a broader focus for the target of abstinence, which members define for themselves with the help of a sponsor. In SLAA, members talk about "bottom-line behaviors" which refer to any behaviors that lead to loss of control in a way that damages the person's life.

Sexaholics Anonymous (SA) is another of the organizations that help adults deal with compulsive sexual behavior. The primary distinction for SA is in the goal of sexual sobriety which SA defines as "having no form of sex with self or with persons" other than a married spouse, with marriage defined as between a man and a woman. Therefore, for a single adult, sexual sobriety is defined as total abstinence.

Sexual Recovery Anonymous (SRA) is most similar to SA in format, but is generally considered to be more flexible in how sexual sobriety is defined, and in the diversity of its membership, with a broader representation of women, people of color, and LGBTQ populations. Family and friends can attend their own peer support groups under the label of "SRA-Anon".

GROUPS FOCUSING ON OTHER BEHAVIORS
Shoplifting can be a compulsive behavior that adults seek peer support in managing. There are local groups that focus on supporting these individuals, as well as a small but growing set of groups in the United States sponsored by the National Association for Shoplifting Prevention (NASP).

Workaholics Anonymous (WA) uses a 12-step format to help members recover from compulsive work. WA has a significant number of phone and on-line meetings, as well as a significant network of in-person meetings in the US and internationally.

GROUPS RELATED TO MEDICAL CONDITIONS (E.G. CANCER, DIABETES, HEART DISEASE, ETC.)

Peer support groups for medical conditions are common, but most are not organized by national or international organizations. They are more commonly associated with local organizations or healthcare providers, and so are more integrated with professional care. This can make them more difficult to locate, as there are fewer easy-to-find listings of groups and locations. You will need to search on-line for local listings by medical condition, or talk with local medical providers.

The lack of large national organizations also means that the format and model used for these groups will vary more widely. Before you refer someone to a group, you may want to do more individual research to find out about how the group works and what it offers participants. Below are a few key categories of medical conditions for which peer support groups are common and growing in popularity.

CANCER

Cancer has a wide variety of forms and can affect children and adults. Stigma is an important issue that people with cancer face, and peer support groups can help address the isolation and other feelings that result from the social stigma. The life threatening nature of some forms of cancer, and the uncertainty that goes along with treatment are also challenges that peer support can help address. Finally, there is a range of treatment navigation and disease self-management challenges that peer support groups can help with. Again, peer support groups are common but not as easy to identify due to the fact that they are often organized within hospitals and healthcare systems. The National Cancer Institute and American Child Cancer Association provide a few of the available listings (see Chapter 15) that can be helpful for identifying groups, but you will want to look for others in your local area.

DEMENTIA AND OTHER NEUROLOGICAL DISORDERS

Alzheimer's Disease and related dementias often create significant strain for the caregivers and family members. The Alzheimer's Association is a national organization that supports a national network of caregiver peer support groups, though there are many local groups affiliated with medical and local non-profits that you may want to search for. Support groups for caregivers of other types of dementia are less common, and many simply attend Alzheimer's caregivers support groups. There has been some development in the area of support groups for those suffering with early dementia(as opposed to caregivers), but this is still in an early phase of development.

<u>Attention Deficit Disorder Association</u> facilitates a series of virtual peer support groups for adults with ADD and for family members. These groups are limited in the times they occur, but because they are virtual, members call in from a range of locations. <u>Children and Adults with Attention-Deficit/Hyperactivity Disorder (CHADD)</u>, is probably the most prominent group providing support to people with ADHD and their family members. CHADD offers a network of peer support groups, though there may be a fee to join a group.

<u>Autism and Asperger's Syndrome</u>: The Global and Regional Asperger's Syndrome Partnerships offers a range of face-to-face and virtual peer support groups, some of which are broad in focus, while others have more focused targets such as parents, family, teens, and LGBT populations.

<u>The Learning Disabilities Association of America (LDAA)</u> is a non-profit organization that includes local affiliates that function as, or can direct individuals to, peer support groups for persons with learning disabilities and/or family members and parents of children with learning disabilities. An example of a web-based international directory of unaffiliated support groups can be found at <u>learndisability.meetup.com</u>, a type of resource that is likely to be more common, and more valuable, as independent peer support groups develop and need to be connected in a way that helps people find them.

<u>The National Multiple Sclerosis Society</u> supports a large network of self-help groups for adults with multiple sclerosis. Many groups are broad in focus, while some are designed for specific

subgroups (e.g. young adults, African-Americans, parents with MS).

Stroke is common and can produce a wide ranging impact on those who experience it. The American Stroke Association, which is an offshoot of the American Heart Association, supports a network of peer support groups across the United States for survivors of stroke. Many groups are linked with local hospital and medical groups, and others are associated with other non-profit or government groups.

Tourette's Syndrome Association provides a directory of peer support groups for those suffering from Tourette's Syndrome and their family members.

Traumatic Brain Injury (TBI) and Concussion are common injuries that have an impact on the person and family and other caregivers. Support groups are available but there is no national organization supporting most, as many are tied to local organizations or healthcare providers.

DIABETES

Diabetes, both type I and type II, are typically chronic illnesses that can be isolating and require significant self-management. Peer support groups can be very helpful in breaking the isolation and helping people develop good self-management skills. There is a wide variety of education and support groups, as well as on-line chat rooms, blogs, and on-line groups providing individual support. The Defeat Diabetes Foundation is one of many sources of information about available peer support groups, including several thousand groups available in the US.

HEART DISEASE

Heart Disease takes many forms, and there is a range of support groups for children and adults who either have heart disease, have had cardiac surgery, and/or are participating in cardiac rehabilitation. There are also support groups for family members and caregivers. Many groups are organized by, or affiliated with local medical resources, but there are several organizations that support networks of support groups.

Mended Hearts is a non-profit network of 300+ "chapters" that meet for peer support, as well as to engage in volunteer service. Mended Hearts has been active since 1952. They partner with hospitals and cardiac rehabilitation centers, and encourage members to reach out to those in care for heart disease through in-person visiting, and phone and email contact. There is a subprogram for children with heart disease called Mended Little Hearts.

WomenHeart: The National Coalition for Women with Heart Disease was founded by three women who had heart attacks while in their 40s and faced challenges in getting treatment and social support. They describe their mission as "to improve the health and quality of life of women living with or at risk of heart disease, and to advocate for their benefit." They support a small but growing network of support groups.

RESPIRATORY PROBLEMS

Respiratory Problems include a number of common illnesses for which there are local and national support group networks. For example, there are support networks for chronic obstructive pulmonary disease (COPD), emphysema, and lung cancer, among others, as well as support groups for those seeking to stop smoking in order to prevent respiratory problems.

OTHER MEDICAL CONDITIONS

Sexually Transmitted Diseases can be associated with significant social stigma, and so peer support groups have an important place in breaking some of the isolation that can be associated with these conditions. The American Sexual Health Association provides a fairly modest listing of some of the active support groups for this group of conditions. The Sexually Transmitted Disease (STD) Project has a more extensive listing of support groups, focusing on supporting adults with Hepatitis.

GROUPS RELATED TO DISABILITIES (E.G. HEARING LOSS, LIMB LOSS, SPINAL CORD INJURY, VISUAL IMPAIRMENT, ETC.)

There are a wide range of support groups for disabled adults and family members of disabled children. They are often organized at a local level. Local chapters of some national organizations support a range of activities, with advocacy typically being more central than peer support. Despite that, here are a sampling of organizations that provide directories of peer support groups.

HEARING LOSS

The Hearing Loss Association of America (HLAA) is an advocacy organization that seeks to provide assistance and resources for people with hearing loss, and their families. HLAA supports chapters in most of the United States, which function as support groups as well as disseminating information and other advocacy work.

LIMB LOSS

The Amputee Coalition of America - National Peer Network (ACA-NPN) is a non-profit organization that seeks to "reach out to and empower people affected by limb loss to achieve their full potential through education, support and advocacy, and to promote limb loss prevention". ACA-NPN provides a directory of 250+ support groups in the United States, most closely affiliated with medical facilities that serve amputees.

SPINAL CORD INJURY
The United Spinal Association provides a national directory of a small but growing number of peer support groups for adults with spinal cord injuries.

VISUAL IMPAIRMENT
The American Foundation for the Blind (AFB) partnered with the Reader's Digest Partners for Sight Foundation to create an on-line resource (VisionAware.com) for visually impaired individuals. This resource includes a growing listing of peer support groups operating in the United States.

Enrichment Audio Resource Service (E.A.R.S.) is a nonprofit organization that maintains a large directory of support groups in the United States for adults with visual impairment seeking to maintain their independence. The directory is called "EARS for EYES".

GROUPS RELATED TO BROADER LIFE CHALLENGES
There has been a remarkable growth in the number and range of peer support groups that have developed around broader life challenges. Many are local, and may be difficult to find without independent research. Here is a sampling of a few that have listings hosted by national organizations.

PEOPLE AFFECTED BY SUICIDE
The American Association of Suicidology (AAS) supports a network of peer support groups for those affected by suicide, including groups for family members and friends of those who

have committed suicide and groups for those who survived suicide attempts.

The American Foundation for Suicide Prevention (AFSP) is another non-profit organization whose work includes helping those affected by suicide. To this end, AFSP supports a network of support groups across the United States.

PEOPLE AFFECTED BY LGBTQ STIGMA

Parents Families and Friends of and Allies United with LGBTQ People (PFLAG) claims to be the largest non-profit organization in the United States committed to advancing equality and full societal affirmation of LGBTQ people. PFLAG has over 400 chapters, many of which appear to function as support and advocacy groups.

Transgender American Veterans Association (TAVA) provides a small but growing directory of support groups for transgender Veterans, providing social support, practical information and advocacy for the challenges faced by this group.

There are many national organizations the focus on advocacy for people affected by LGBTQ stigma. While they also provide social support, there are also local organizations that provide support groups and a range of other forms of support for people affected by LGBTQ stigma. Searching for local groups will likely be one of the best strategies for finding support groups in your area.

PEOPLE AFFECTED BY SEXUAL IDENTITY ISSUES

Again, searching for local organizations that provide and sponsor support groups for individuals looking for support around sexual identity, medical conditions that impact sexual identity, stigma related to sexual identity, and related issues, may be your best strategy to find support that is available near you.

Intersex Society of North America (ISNA) is one example of a national group that does provide some information about support opportunities. ISNA defines "intersex" as a status resulting from various "conditions in which a person is born with a reproductive or sexual anatomy that doesn't seem to fit the typical definitions of female or male." ISNA is a good source of information on a diverse network of support groups organized through various organizations supporting people who are intersex due to a number of specific causes.

PEOPLE AFFECTED BY LOSS AND BEREAVEMENT

The Compassionate Friends provide a network of peer support groups for family members who have lost a child. There are at least 600 peer support groups across the United States.

Tragedy Assistance Program for Survivors (TAPS) is a non-profit organization that supports anyone grieving the death of a loved one who died while serving in the United States military. Among other forms of 1-1 and educational support, TAPS supports a relatively small network of peer-support groups in about 15 states, as well as on-line support.

CHALLENGES RELATED TO PARENTING

Parents Anonymous is a non-profit organization whose mission of strengthening families also seeks to help families prevent child abuse. Among other education and advocacy services, Parents Anonymous supports a network of weekly adult groups and children and youth groups. These groups seek to "offer a caring and supportive environment where parents and caregivers support each other and explore new parenting strategies, address underlying emotional issues, and create long lasting positive changes in their families." Groups are co-led by a parent leader and a facilitator, and use content developed by the organization.

Because I Love You, is a non-profit organization that supports a small but growing network of peer support groups in the United States and Canada for parents who have children (of all ages) with behavioral issues such as substance use, truancy, and verbal and physical acting out.

Mothers of Twins Clubs, aka Multiples of America (Twins, Triplets etc.) provide support for parents, and expectant parents of twins and other multiple births. This non-profit supports a network of over 200 clubs around the United States.

Attachment Parenting International (API) is an example of the growing number of organizations developing peer support groups for parents seeking to establish healthy patterns of parenting, or to repair damaged relationships within their families.   Like many of these groups, API has a specific model of healthy parenting that is promoted through a network of parent support groups that are active primarily in the US, but some of which exist in other countries.

Parents Without Partners (PWP) describes itself as the largest non-profit organization supporting single parents and their children, with the goal of providing opportunities for enhancing personal growth, self-confidence and sensitivity towards others. They have a relatively small but growing number of chapters in the U.S. and Canada, which have a variety of functions, including acting as support groups.

Resolve (The National Infertility Association) is a non-profit organization focusing on improving the lives of women and men impacted by infertility. They support a national network of support groups in the United States, most of which appear to be peer-led, though some groups are professionally led.

PEOPLE EXPERIENCING TRAUMA

Support groups for victims of crime are often organized at a local level. You may want to look at your local state or regional government, including offices of state attorneys general for listings of support groups. National organizations typically have a primary mission of advocacy, but some do have support groups.

Mothers Against Drunk Driving (MADD) has support groups for those affected by the actions of drunk drivers. They do not list their groups in a national directory, but you can check with your local chapter.

Parents of Murdered Children (POMC) is similar to MADD, in that they support victim groups as part of their mission, but you will need to contact your local chapter to see what is available in your area.

Victims of Domestic Violence can benefit from peer support groups to address the wide range of challenges they experience. You will need to look for local sources of information about peer support groups, as there is limited information posted nationally, in part due to the need to protect visibility of some victims for their safety. Similarly, support groups for Victims of Sexual Assault are common, but national listings are not. You may want to talk with local clinicians about making a referral and strategies for finding active groups.

PEOPLE AFFECTED BY CHALLENGES RELATED TO EMPLOYMENT

<u>Unemployment</u> is associated with a great deal of social stigma that can be addressed in part by peer support groups. <u>Searching for Employment</u> is often a highly stressful task that can be helped by peer support. There is a wide array of support groups for those who are unemployed and those looking for employment. Some are organized by local and regional governmental employment services. Others are totally independent, though many government (national, regional, local) labor offices can help you find them (for example, see your local Department of Labor <u>CareerOneStops</u>, now called <u>American Job Centers</u>, for assistance in finding job clubs or other groups).

There are national listings that may be helpful. <u>JobHunt.org</u> is an example of a national job hunting resource website that includes a large listing of support-networking groups around the United States. Regional networks are more common, and will require some searching. For example, <u>Neighbors-Helping-Neighbors</u> is an example of a job search and networking organization which hosts meetings that mix the provision of support with networking for those looking for employment in the New Jersey-New York area, though it is growing beyond that area.

GROUPS SERVING 'AT-RISK' POPULATIONS

Many people work in jobs or roles that are associated with special stressors or challenges that would benefit from peer support. Examples include first responders, members of the military, Veterans, some groups of healthcare providers, and those at elevated risk for some illnesses. This is an area of rapid growth in peer support, most of it happening at the local level with limited national organization. To help find support groups, you will need to talk with people in those groups or local organizations that support those people.

CHAPTER 14

LEGAL AND ETHICAL ISSUES

As a peer support group leader, you will need to know about legal and ethical issues related to self-help groups and your role as leader. If you work within a larger organization, or are leading a support group affiliated with a larger organization, your best source of guidance will be the organization itself. Most will have specific guidelines and expectations that reflect the legal and ethical issues they feel you need to attend to. Get to know these guidelines and follow them. Also, talk about the guidelines with supervisors and colleagues. Your understanding will help you avoid unpleasant situations.

This chapter is designed to point out some of the common legal or ethical issues related to peer support groups. It is beyond the scope of this chapter to do a thorough review of legal and ethical issues. I am not aware of anyone who has done this in written form, and I am not a lawyer and thus not qualified to do so. The limited extent of explicit legal guidance available for peer support groups reflects the fact that there have been limited legal guidelines established. This is slowly changing, and so this chapter highlights some of the emerging issues in an attempt to raise awareness of them.

LEGAL ISSUES

Because peer support groups are composed of adults who freely choose to come together to support each other, there is relatively less opening for legal concerns relative to groups run by clinical providers. The basic assumption is that anyone attending a self-help group is choosing to come and so is responsible for that choice. As leader, you are helping to support the meeting, but have limited responsibility for what happens between the adults who attend. Yet, even in this type of arrangement, there are a few potential problems that can come up, and it is important to highlight those and talk about some strategies that have been taken by some organizations to address them.

Confused Expectations. Peer support/self-help groups are by definition distinct from groups that represent clinical interventions led by licensed professionals. In clinical groups, the leader is highly accountable for what he or she does, having to meet legal and ethical guidelines established by laws, professional standards, and other guidelines. Peer support groups, and by extension peer support group leaders, also have to meet some expectations, albeit much less demanding expectations than those for a service offered by a clinician.

It is possible that some peer support group attendees may not be clear on what kind of group they are participating in, and so might mistakenly think that your meeting is a clinical intervention such as group psychotherapy, and that you are a licensed clinician. You want to ensure that no one coming to the group misunderstands the nature of the group or your role. To do that, you want to think about how you can effectively educate people and how you can show that they actually understand what you have told them.

A few simple steps have been taken by some organizations to ensure there is no confusion.

- Some organizations include a review of the nature of the group at the beginning of each meeting. Most groups have some form of standard introduction, and so it can be helpful to include some consistent language about the fact that this is a peer support group that involves people coming together to support each other.
- Some organizations expect notes or a summary of each meeting to be created and saved. In that case, it can be helpful to include in that documentation that you started the meeting with this type of reminder about the nature of the group.
- Some organizations interview anyone who wants to join the group before they start attending. This is a good opportunity to ensure that prospective members understand the nature of the group and all of the expectations of participation. In some cases, prospective members are asked to sign a document at the end of this initial interview, noting that they understand the expectations of the group, and that this a peer support group.
- You will want to avoid acting in any way that would suggest you are a clinician. For example, be careful not to give medical or healthcare advice as though you have clinical expertise. You may, however, have expertise in participating in healthcare from the patient's perspective and commenting about your experience can be very helpful. But if you make recommendations as though you are a clinician or an expert in clinical care, it can lead people to be confused about your credentials—and to increased liability for you.

Injury and Harm to Participants. Though it is rare, bad things can happen to people at peer support groups. These include the following:

- Attendees can have simple accidents before, during, or after the meeting in which they get hurt. For example, someone could be injured during a meeting by tripping over an electric cord stretched across the floor.

- Attendees could suffer physical or emotional harm before, during, or after the meeting as a result of some action by them or another attendee.

- Attendees may be harmed by someone in the group sharing confidential comments with a third party outside the group.

- Attendees can become involved with other people in the group who are dangerous in some way, and then through that relationship can be harmed. There has been some national attention to cases in which criminals who were required to attend 12-step groups (as part of a legal proceeding) victimized other members in the group.

While peer support organizations and leaders cannot be held responsible for all of the bad things that can happen to people who attend a peer support group, there is increasing attention paid to reducing the risk of harm, and how to address legal liability.

- Liability Insurance: Some organizations that support or sponsor peer support groups have started to require that chapters carry liability insurance to protect against legal claims of injury. This is similar to homeowners insurance that protects the group against a lawsuit from anyone who may be accidentally injured during participation. Some of the community organizations that allow peer support groups to meet at their facilities (e.g., churches/synagogues/temples/mosques, schools, businesses) are now requiring that chapters/groups have liability insurance before they use their facility. You will want to inquire with your organization whether this applies to the group you are leading. If your group is held at a clinical facility, it is likely that they already have liability coverage, though it would be worth discussing with them.

- It is also important to note that liability issues can extend to <u>transporting members</u> to groups. Some organizations have asked group leaders not to transport members to meetings in an effort to avoid liability for any injuries that might occur during transportation. You'll want to talk with your organization about this topic and think about how you want to deal with this liability issue.

- <u>Informed Consent</u>: Because some of the risks involved in participating in peer support groups are inherent in the activity, one of the strategies used to protect leaders and members is to educate them about the risks before they participate. For example, most groups have guidelines about keeping comments made in the group confidential. Some groups inform all prospective members about this rule, but also add the limitation that the group and group leader cannot guarantee that all members will always follow this rule, and that attendees should keep this in mind when they are choosing what to say. Those groups that have prospective members participate in a screening interview may want to review this point at that time, and even include it in a statement signed by the prospective members, showing that they understand the risk they are taking. Similarly, participation in peer support groups can lead to upsetting discussions. It may be useful to inform prospective members of this fact and even include it in their signed consent.

- <u>Protections for Confidentiality</u>: It is reasonable to expect that peer support group leaders recognize the value of confidentiality for group members and take basic steps to protect it. For example, besides regularly reminding members about the importance of confidentiality, group leaders should be attentive to the potential problems created when the group creates and circulates lists of members. Those lists can find their way outside the group and break expectations of privacy. Similarly, distributing photos and email lists can lead to outside people finding out about who is participating in a group. Simple steps such as asking members to sign waivers before lists, emails, or photos are shared can ensure everyone is making a conscious decision about privacy. Similarly, simply trying to minimize situations in which confidentiality can be compromised, and talking about these with all group members, can help reduce the risk of bad situations.

- <u>Expectation of Reasonable Actions of the Group Leader to Address Risk</u>: As a peer support group leader, you are not held to the same standard as a clinician in terms of protecting participants. However, it is often helpful to think of what is reasonable for the community, and your group members, to expect from you in terms of what you should do to respond to dangers that you see. If you see a member who seems to be dangerous to other members in some clear way, is it reasonable to expect that you would take action to try to protect the group? It is unclear what the legal system expects, but some organizations that sponsor peer support groups are being increasingly explicit about the expectation that group leaders are to take action to address clear dangers to group members. This expectation is mostly regarding dangers represented by other members who either (1) have such behavior problems that they could hurt other members or (2) have such criminal or predatory behavior problems that they are likely to victimize other members. In its 2014 guidelines for peer support group leaders, the National Multiple Sclerosis Society explicitly states that it is in everyone's interest to actively deal with the rare situations in which a member's disruptive behavior and/or mistreatment of other members threatens the group. They rightly point out that the group leader is responsible for taking action in these situations, but should not act alone. The leader should involve the organization, supervisors, and colleagues in any decisions and actions.

- It is important to note that these situations are rare. However, you will want to think through how you might deal with them in case they do arise. More importantly, you will want to talk with your sponsoring organization, your supervisor, your mentor, and your colleagues about what they are doing or would do. If a situation arises where you think a reasonable risk is present, you want to contact these other parties immediately to get their direction and support. In those situations, you may want to document that you got this advice or guidance, either by keeping any electronic or written records of the guidance, or by summarizing the discussion in an email that you send to yourself and keep.

Harm or Risk of Harm to Others Outside the Group. It is possible, though unlikely, that someone in your group might make a comment during your meeting that indicates that this person either has hurt others or is planning to hurt others outside your group. Depending on the nature of the comment, licensed clinicians and other professionals have legal, ethical, or organizational requirements to take action in those situations, either to ensure the safety of others or to ensure law enforcement knows about illegal activity. This is particularly true if the comments indicate that children, disabled, or elderly people have been abused, or that significant violence is likely to happen to a specific person.

You do not have the same external requirements, but you should consider what a reasonable response would be to comments that group members make. Again, you will want to talk with your sponsoring organization, your supervisor, your mentor, and your colleagues about what they want you to do, or would advise you to do. In these situations, you will want to contact others quickly to get their input. Making a decision about a responsible action tends to be easier with input from others. Sometimes, people feel conflicted about taking an action that might break the group's confidentiality. While this is understandable, you want to be aware that you are weighing confidentiality versus the safety of someone. In most cases in which there is a real risk of abuse or violence, the safety of a child or vulnerable adult is going to be more important than the confidentiality of your group.

If, after talking with your organization and respected colleagues, you decide that action is warranted to protect someone's safety, be aware that you should not directly intervene (e.g., you should not go to someone's home to stop violence). If you feel you need to take some form of action, you will again want to draw in colleagues to help activate the professional providers who will take action. These include clinical providers, social service agencies, and the police. They have the training and responsibility for intervening—your job is just to inform them of the situation and let them do their job.

To help address such a situation before it even arises, and to ensure that members are thoughtful about what they share in the group, some peer support groups include information in an informed consent form or comfort agreement about what may happen if members make comments to the group about having hurt or planning to hurt others. If you will respond in any predictable way to those types of comments (e.g., calling child protective agencies if a member reports abusing children), you may want to include this in the information you share with all prospective members.

Financial Concerns. Peer support groups are almost always free to participants, which limits the issues that arise when money is involved. Some peer support groups raise funds, which they use for various projects that support the mission of the group. Whenever money is involved, the opportunity for illegal and unethical behavior by someone in the group can arise. Again, talk with your larger organization and with other peer group leaders about how they deal with financial concerns and what steps they routinely take to guard against misuse of funds. They will likely have specific suggestions that you will want to follow.

Liability Concerns of Those Referring to Self-Help Groups. There has been some discussion of whether there is any liability for those who refer people to a peer support group if something goes wrong at the group. A recent published review concluded the liability risk for referral sources is "small" (Salzer & Kundra, 2010) and is linked to whether the referral source knew of significant problems in the group they were referring to.

One of the few issues that referral sources should be aware of is the issue of referral to religious versus non-religious peer groups. Government agencies that mandate attendance at self-help groups have been given guidance that they cannot mandate referral to religious groups alone, but need to include the option for a non-religious support group as well. Many people, for example, either feel uncomfortable at 12-step groups or don't attend them because they don't agree with the religious content. A number of organizations sponsor groups that are neutral about religion. Referral sources, including peer group leaders, will better serve those they are referring by attending to their feelings about groups with religious content, and ensuring they know about religion-neutral options (see chapter 13 for examples).

ETHICAL ISSUES

As a self-help group leader, the way you conduct yourself in terms of ethical behavior will help you avoid a wide range of problems. You must work in accordance with the ethical guidelines established by any organization you serve. Here is a list of additional common ethical guidelines for people providing peer support services.

- Maintain high standards of personal conduct.
- Support the self-determination of the group members and potential group members you work with.
- Respect the rights and dignity of all group members and potential group members, including their right to privacy and confidentiality.
- Respect individual and cultural differences of group members and potential group members. Never practice or condone any form of discrimination.
- Never intimidate, threaten, harass, or use excessive influence, physical force, or verbal abuse against group members and potential group members.
- Never engage in sexual or intimate activities with members of a group you lead.

CHAPTER 15

YOUR RESOURCE LIST

This section is divided into two sections, the first serving as a general list of the resources you may need to support those you are assisting. The second section consists of a series of tables providing links to national and regional directories of peer support groups, with room for you to add additional regional and local links that you and your colleagues may be interested in.

These tables are designed to help you, your colleagues, and your clients to quickly contact people or organizations that may be useful. To be most helpful, take some time to fill in those contacts that are specific to your position, setting, organization, and regional area. This may take some initial research, and some effort to keep it up to date, but the resulting resource list will be a very handy tool that you will use many times.

PART I: QUICK REFERENCE CONTACTS:

CONTACT	PHONE NUMBERS	EMAIL
Local Police		
Local Fire Dept.		
Local Emergency Room(s)		
Suicide Prevention Hotline		
Child Abuse Hotline		
Elder Abuse Hotline		
Rape Hotline		
Intimate Partner/Domestic Violence Resource		
Pregnancy Resource		
Poison Control Hotline		

Local Homelessness/ Housing Resource		
In Your Organization		
Your "Supervisor":		
Other Contacts:		
Other Contacts:		
Other Peer Support/Self-Help Group Leaders		

Other Common Referral Resources		
Outpatient Mental Health Svc.		
Case Management		
Vocational Services		
Housing Services		
Religious or Spiritual Counseling		
Benefits Counseling		
Local Clubhouse or Consumer Run Organization		

PART II: A SAMPLING OF DIRECTORIES OF OTHER PEER SUPPORT GROUP RESOURCES

Please note that this list is meant only as a sample listing of the range of peer support resources available in the community. You will likely want to look for the larger set of available group resources for the people you are serving, searching both online and through personal contacts for those local and regional groups that are active in your area.

The listings below are in no way an endorsement of these organizations or of the specific self-help groups they are listing. In most situations, you will want to investigate individual groups to see if they are active and whether they have a reputation that supports your referral.

The listings are organized by category of service. You'll notice that blank lines have been included for you to add additional listings for groups that you find out about and that you may want to refer others to.

TABLE IIA: GROUPS RELATED TO THE MISUSE OF DRUGS AND ALCOHOL

CONDITION/ ORGANIZATION	DIRECTORY OF SUPPORT GROUPS
Alcoholics Anonymous (AA)	http://www.aa.org/pages/en_US/find-aa-resources
Al-Anon	http://www.al-anon.org/find-a-meeting
Alateen	http://al-anon.info/MeetingSearch/AlateenMeetings.aspx?language=EN
Cocaine Anonymous (CA)	http://www.ca.org/meetings.html
Crystal Meth Anonymous (CMA):	http://www.crystalmeth.org/cma-meeting.html
Dual Recovery Anonymous	http://www.draonline.org/meetings.html
Families Anonymous In US:

International: | http://www.familiesanonymous.org/index.php?route=information/information&information_id=22

http://www.familiesanonymous.org/index.php?route=information/information&information_id=23 |
Life Ring Secular Recovery (LRSR)	http://lifering.org/find-a-meeting/
Marijuana Anonymous (MA)	https://www.marijuana-anonymous.org/meetings/find
Moderation Management (MM)	http://www.moderation.org/meetings/index.shtml
Narcotics Anonymous (NA)	http://www.na.org/meetingsearch/

Nar-Anon	http://www.nar-anon.org/find-a-meeting/
Nicotine Anonymous	https://nicotine-anonymous.org/find-a-meeting.html
Secular Organization for Sobriety (SOS)	http://www.sossobriety.org/meetings.html
SMART Recovery	http://www.smartrecovery.org/meetings_db/view/
Women for Sobriety (WFS)	http://womenforsobriety.org/beta2/group-info/

TABLE IIB: GROUPS RELATED TO BROADER MENTAL HEALTH CONDITIONS (E.G. DEPRESSION, ANXIETY, BIPOLAR DISORDER, SCHIZOPHRENIA)

CONDITION/ ORGANIZATION	DIRECTORY OF SUPPORT GROUPS
Anxiety and Depression Assoc. of America (ADAA)	http://www.adaa.org/finding-help/getting-support/support-groups
Attention Deficit Disorder Association	https://add.org/adhd-support-groups/
Depression Bipolar Support Alliance (DBSA)	http://www.dbsalliance.org/site/PageServer?pagename=peer_support_group_locator
Depressed Anonymous (DA)	http://www.depressedanon.com/
Dialectical Behavior Therapy (DBT) Peer Support Groups	http://dialectical-behavior-therapy-dbt.meetup.com/
Dual Recovery Anonymous	http://www.draonline.org/meetings.html
Emotions Anonymous (EA)	http://allone.com/12/ea/
Gift From Within	http://www.giftfromwithin.org/html/groups.html
International Obsessive Compulsive Foundation	https://iocdf.org/find-help/

National Alliance on Mental Illness (NAMI): Peer groups, family groups	https://www.nami.org/Local-NAMI/Programs?classkey=39d47f5e- https://www.nami.org/Find-Support https://www.nami.org/Local-NAMI/Programs?classkey=1d79b22b-d10a-43fe-8ab7-ede96c824fa8
Postpartum Progress	http://www.postpartumprogress.com/ppd-support-groups-in-the-u-s-canada
Postpartum Support International	http://www.postpartum.net/get-help/locations/united-states/
Recovery International / The Abraham Low Institute (RI/TALI)	https://www.recoveryinternational.org/meetings/find-a-meeting/
Schizophrenics Anonymous (SA)	http://www.sardaa.org/sa-group-locations/
Wellness Recovery Action Plan (WRAP) Support Groups	Look for regional listings such as: http://recoveringnancy.weebly.com/wrap-support-groups.html

TABLE IIC: GROUPS RELATED TO TROUBLING BEHAVIORS (E.G. DISORDERED EATING, GAMBLING OR SEX)

CONDITION/ ORGANIZATION	DIRECTORY OF SUPPORT GROUPS
Anorexics and Bulimics Anonymous (ABA)	http://aba12steps.org/aba-meetings/meetings/
Bettors Anonymous	http://www.bettorsanonymous.org/meeting.html
Debtors Anonymous (DA)	http://www.debtorsanonymous.org/admin/index.php/find
Eating Disorders Anonymous	http://www.eatingdisordersanonymous.org/meetings.html
Gamblers Anonymous (GA)	http://www.gamblersanonymous.org/ga/locations
National Association for Shoplifting Prevention	http://www.shopliftingprevention.org/local-self-help-groups/
National Eating Disorders Association	http://www.nationaleatingdisorders.org/find-help-support
Overeaters Anonymous (OA)	https://www.oa.org/membersgroups/group-support/
Sex Addicts Anonymous (SAA)	https://saa-recovery.org/Meetings/
Sexual Compulsives Anonymous (SCA)	http://www.sca-recovery.org/find.htm#online
Sex and Love Addicts Anonymous (SLAA)	http://www.slaafws.org/meetings
Sexaholics Anonymous (SA)	http://www.sa.org/meetings.php

Sexual Recovery Anonymous (SRA)	http://www.sexualrecovery.org/find_a_meeting.html
Workaholics Anonymous (WA)	http://www.workaholics-anonymous.org/meetings/wa-meetings

TABLE IID: GROUPS RELATED TO OTHER MEDICAL CONDITIONS (E.G. CANCER, DIABETES, HEART DISEASE, NEUROLOGIC DISORDERS, ETC.)

CONDITION/ ORGANIZATION	DIRECTORY OF SUPPORT GROUPS
CANCER	
American Childhood Cancer Association	http://www.acco.org/groups/local-groups/
National Cancer Institute	http://supportorgs.cancer.gov/searchresults.aspx?sid=hXr7lTFUtQJjYqnn6brmJAXCQBb5CNYFQNoKj02M%2BrI%3D
Lung Cancer Alliance	http://www.lungcanceralliance.org/get-help-and-support/coping-with-lung-cancer/support-groups/
Cancer.net	http://www.cancer.net/coping-with-cancer/finding-support-and-information/general-cancer-groups
DEMENTIA AND OTHER NEUROLOGICAL DISORDERS	
Alzheimer's Disease and Related Dementias	http://www.alz.org/care/alzheimers-dementia-support-groups.asp#group
Attention Deficit Disorder (ADD/ADHD)	http://www.chadd.org/
Autism and Asperger's Syndrome	http://grasp.org/page/grasp-support-groups

Learning Disabilities Association of America	http://ldaamerica.org/support/state-local-affiliates/
Learndisability.meet up.com	http://learndisability.meetup.com/
National Multiple Sclerosis Society	http://www.nationalmssociety.org/Resources-Support/Find-Support/Join-a-Local-Support-Group
Stroke	http://www.strokeassociation.org/STROKEORG/strokegroup/public/zipFinder.jsp for a resource booklet: http://www.strokeassociation.org/STROKEORG/LifeAfterStroke/FindingSupportYouAreNotAlone/Stroke-Support-Group
Tourette's Syndrome Association	http://tourette.org/AboutUs/usa_chp_sup_cofe.html
DIABETES	
Defeat Diabetes Foundation	http://www.defeatdiabetes.org/our-community/business-directory/list/adult-diabetes-support-groups/

HEART DISEASE	
Mended Hearts	https://mendedhearts.gnosishosting.net/Chapters
WomenHeart	http://www.womenheart.org/?page=Support_Networks

RESPIRATORY ILLNESS	
COPD & Emphysema	http://www.lung.org/support-and-community/better-breathers-club/
Lung Cancer Alliance	http://www.lungcanceralliance.org/get-help-and-support/coping-with-lung-cancer/support-groups/

OTHER MEDICAL CONDITIONS	
Herpes, Hepatitis, HIV	http://www.ashasexualhealth.org/stdsstis/herpes/support-groups/ http://www.thestdproject.com/std-resources/hepatitis-support-groups-by-location/

TABLE IIE: GROUPS RELATED TO DISABILITIES (E.G. HEARING IMPAIRMENT LIMB LOSS, SPINAL CORD INJURY, VISUAL IMPAIRMENT, ETC.)

CONDITION/ ORGANIZATION	DIRECTORY OF SUPPORT GROUPS
HEARING IMPAIRMENT	
Hearing Impaired	http://www.hearingloss.org/support_resources/find-local-hlaa-chapter
LIMB LOSS	
National Amputee Coalition	http://www.amputee-coalition.org/support-groups-peer-support/support-group-network/
SPINL CORD INJURY	
SpinalCord.org	http://www.spinalcord.org/spinal-network/support-groups/
Wheel of Life	http://wheel-life.org/connecting-peer-support-group-community/

VISUAL IMPAIRMENT	
VisionAware.org	http://www.visionaware.org/directory. aspx?action=results&CategoryID=104
EARS for EYES	http://www.earsforeyes.info/ears/tblLi nkslist.php
OTHER DISABILITY	

TABLE IIF: GROUPS RELATED TO
BROADER LIFE CHALLENGES

CONDITION/ ORGANIZATION	DIRECTORY OF SUPPORT GROUPS
PEOPLE AFFECTED BY SUICIDE	
American Association of Suicidology (AAS)	http://www.suicidology.org/suicide-survivors/sos-directory
American Foundation for Suicide Prevention	http://www.afsp.org/coping-with-suicide-loss/find-support/find-a-support-group
PEOPLE AFFECTED BY LGBTQ STIGMA	
PFLAG	http://pflag-chapter-map.herokuapp.com/
TAVA	http://transveteran.org/for-veterans/trans-support-locator/
PEOPLE AFFECTED BY GENDER IDENTITY ISSUES	
Intersex	http://www.isna.org/support

PEOPLE AFFECTED BY LOSS AND BEREAVEMENT	
Compassionate Friends	http://www.compassionatefriends.org/Find_Support/Chapters/Chapter_Locator.aspx
Mended Hearts	https://mendedhearts.gnosishosting.net/Chapters
TAPS	http://www.taps.org/survivors/caregroups.aspx

PEOPLE AFFECTED BY PARENTING ISSUES	
Parents Anonymous	http://parentsanonymous.org/programs/parents-anonymous-groups/network-map/
Because I Love You	http://www.bily.org/helping-parents/locations/
Multiples of America (Parents of Twins etc.)	http://www.multiplesofamerica.org/find-a-club/
Attachment Parenting International (API)	http://www.attachmentparenting.org/groups
Parents Without Partners	http://www.parentswithoutpartners.org/?page=FindChapter
Resolve (That National Infertility Association)	http://www.resolve.org/support/support-group/support-groups-list.html

PEOPLE AFFECTED BY ISSUES RELATED TO EMPLOYMENT	
Dept. of Labor: Career One Source (American Job Centers)	Job Club Listing: http://www.servicelocator.org/national_l ocators.asp?cat=job+club
JobHunt.org	http://www.job-hunt.org/job-search-networking/job-search-networking.shtml#cat1169
Neighbors Helping Neighbors	http://www.nhnusa.org/index.html

APPENDIX A: A BRIEF SUMMARY OF RESEARCH FINDINGS ABOUT PEER SUPPORT GROUPS

There may be times when you will want or need to talk about the evidence from published research studies regarding the benefits of peer support groups. While there are many questions that have not been well-researched, there are many studies of peer support groups that give you helpful information for talking with clinicians, and others. It is important to note that the vast majority of research that has been done, has focused on AA and other 12-step peer support groups. When you talk with others about these results, it is important to note that limitation. However, it is worth noting as well, that for most questions, the answers coming from studies of 12-step peer support groups are likely to be very relevant to other peer support groups.

CONCLUSION	RESEARCH ARTICLES
Participation in peer support/self-help groups is enormous and growing. • In the US, there are more visits to self-help groups than to specialty mental health providers. • Almost 20% of Americans have attended at least one self-help group, and at least 7% have done so in the prior year. • Rates of participation have been growing steadily.	Kessler et al., 1997

Participation in AA and NA is associated with significantly higher rates of abstinence from using drugs and alcohol.	Kaskutas, 2009 Humphreys, 2004
Participation in other peer support groups focusing on mental health/social issues is associated with improvement in the target outcome including: • Overall mental health. • Depression. • Social support.	Marmar et al., 1988 Bright et al., 1999 Houlston et al., 2011
Some initial research findings suggest that participation in other peer support groups focusing on physical health can be associated with improvements in: • Confidence and coping. • Self-care. • Energy. • Social Support. • Pain. • Blood pressure. • Mental Health, Depression. • Communication with Physicians. • Diet. • Exercise and Relaxation. *It is important to note that the formats of the interventions that were studied varied widely, and these results should be considered cautiously.*	Kennedy et al., 2007 Schulz et al., 2008 Griffiths et al., 2005 Barlow et al., 2000

Participation in peer support groups for family members of people with mental illness is associated with improved mental health for the family member and support and improved outcome for the relative with mental illness	Chien et al., 2008 Heller et al., 1997
The size of the benefit of participation in peer support groups for substance use or mental health problems is similar to the size of benefit resulting from participating in clinical care for alcohol use.	Bright et al., 1999 Marmar et al., 1988
Most people who attend AA or other peer support groups, also receive formal care for the issue they are seeking help with.	Kessler et al., 1997
Participation in clinical programs along with AA is associated with better outcomes than participation in clinical programs alone.	Pagano et al., 2013 Kelly et al., 2010 Moos & Moos, 2005
Participation in self-help groups may reduce the cost of healthcare.	Humphreys et al., 2007
Clinical programs that actively refer their patients to peer-support groups, have better clinical outcomes.	Litt et al, 2009 Walitzer et al., 2009 Timko et al., 2006
Clinical providers' efforts to use specific strategies to encourage their patients/clients to participate in peer support groups result in better attendance. These successful strategies include: • Raising the topic with patients and verbally encouraging participation. • Providing written information about specific peer support groups (location, directions, time). • Arranging for a support group member to meet or to call a patient to talk about the	Timko et al, 2011 Walitzer et al., 2009

group. • Asking for a verbal or written commitment from the patient to attend a meeting. • Following up after a referral to a peer support group, by asking about attendance and encouraging participation.	
Some of the specific benefits of peer support groups include: • Increasing positive social support. • Reducing social connections that encourage drinking or other negative behavior. • Improving coping skills. • Improving confidence. • Improving mental health.	Humphreys et al., 1999 Kaskutas et al., 2002 Tonigan et al., 2009 Kelly et al., 2011
Internet-based peer support groups have positive benefits that are similar to in-person support groups.	Riper et al, 2011 Houston et al., 2002

APPENDIX B: DEALING WITH CRITICAL SITUATIONS

As a facilitator of a peer support/self-help group, you will be in situations where you may have to respond to a range of high-risk challenges. Knowing how to respond effectively is essential for all peer support group leaders, regardless of where you work and what your particular focus might be.

BROAD STRATEGIES

- Learn and follow the local guidelines for emergency responses at your organization. Talk about them with your supervisor so you are clear on all procedures before emergencies happen.

- Practice response procedures so you know them fully. Practice and preparation before an incident will ensure that you know how to respond well when a true emergency arises, and that you can do so while under stress.

- Alert others immediately when you find yourself in an emergency situation. Activate safety alert systems and notify other co-workers. Clinical providers have special training in dealing with clinical emergencies. Get them involved quickly and let them take the lead.

- Try to stay calm. Your ability to think clearly will be critical for following through with an effective response.

- "First things first": Attend to immediate safety needs for yourself and those around you before placing all your attention elsewhere.

MAKING A 911 CALL

- Tell the operator what and where the emergency is.

- If someone is injured, tell the operator who is injured and the nature of the injury.

- If there are ongoing dangers in the area that could affect the responders, describe these for the operator.

- Give your name and phone number.

- Do <u>not</u> hang up until instructed to do so by the operator.

- After the call, notify your supervisor and/or other key personnel.

- Make sure someone meets the responders and guides them to the appropriate location.

- Do <u>not</u> move injured people unless it is absolutely necessary. If medical providers are available, let them decide whether to move anyone who has been hurt or administer other emergency first aid.

- Let the responders do their job once they arrive.

- Document your actions.

- After the event is over, talk with your supervisor and co-workers about how the response went and how it could be better next time.

A POTENTIALLY SUICIDAL CLIENT

Suicide is one of the top ten causes of death in the United States, and having a mental health or substance use disorder is one of the most powerful predictors of suicide, suicide attempts, and suicidal thoughts. Peer support group leaders are very likely to have contact with people who are suicidal, and so will want to seek out training and supervisor guidance on how to deal with this common and critical situation.

If you think someone may be suicidal, contact your supervisor or another available clinician as quickly as possible. Clinical providers often have significant training in assessing and responding to suicidal adults. Get them involved quickly and follow their guidance.

However, it's not always easy to know if a client is suicidal. Someone may need to ask the person for more information before it becomes clear that he or she is at risk. Talk with your supervisor about whether you should notify them immediately or first ask questions of the client directly on your own.

Watch for some of the following common warning signs:

- Talking about suicide.

- Getting the means to commit suicide.

- Being preoccupied with death.

- Withdrawing from social contact; wanting to be left alone.

- Feeling trapped or hopeless.

- Engaging in risky or self-destructive behaviors.

- Increasing substance abuse.

- Giving away belongings; getting affairs in order for death.

If you are going to speak with the client before seeking out a supervisor or other clinician, ask clear simple questions:

- "Do you feel like giving up?"

- "Do you think a lot about dying?"

- "Have you been having thoughts about hurting yourself?"

- "Have you thought about how you might hurt yourself?"

- "Do you have the means of hurting yourself available to you?"

If you believe the client is actively suicidal:

- Do not leave them alone—stay engaged with them.

- Get help as quickly as possible. Call a supervisor, 911 or the police, depending on how critical the situation is and who is immediately available to you.

- Keep the person engaged while help is coming.

- Encourage the person to get help.

- Offer to go with the person to get help.

- Be respectful of their feelings. Don't be judgmental or patronizing.

A POTENTIALLY HOMICIDAL OR VIOLENT CLIENT

Violence occurs in many work settings, including mental health settings. Training and preparation are critical for recognizing potential risks and preventing violent incidents.

If you think someone has the potential for violence in the near future, contact your supervisor or another available clinician immediately. Again, clinical providers typically have significant training in assessing and responding to potential violence. Get them involved quickly.

It's not always easy to recognize if someone has the potential to be violent in the near future. That's why it is important to take the following common precautions in all settings.

- If you work in a specific area, think about how to make the area safer. For example, make sure you have a way to leave safely if someone becomes threatening. Keep the space relatively uncluttered—eliminate items that someone could use to hurt you or others.

- Have ways to get help quickly, and know how to use them (e.g. panic buttons or alarms).

- Talk with co-workers and supervisors in your area about how you can work together to respond to a potentially violent situation.

- Know how to access security and police officials quickly. Talk with them about working together for safety.

- Request a formal assessment of safety by a licensed professional.

A SITUATION THAT INVOLVES POSSIBLE "INTIMATE PARTNER VIOLENCE" OR "DOMESTIC ABUSE"

Intimate partner violence (IPV) refers to physical or sexual violence, threats, or emotional abuse between people who have or have had an intimate relationship. Accurate data about IPV is difficult to collect, but at least 30% of women and 10% of men will experience IPV in their lifetimes.

Learn and follow the local guidelines for responding to these situations. Talk about them with your supervisor before you uncover actual situations and have to respond.

If you think you are working with someone involved in a violent relationship, or if you think it is likely there is violence, contact your supervisor or another available clinician as quickly as possible. As stated before, clinical providers often have significant training in identifying, assessing, and responding to violence.

It's often not easy to tell if someone is experiencing IPV, and many people are hesitant to talk about it. Watch for some of the most common warning signs that may identify victims of IPV:

- They appear overly afraid of or anxious to please their partner.

- They may talk about their partner's temper or possessive or controlling nature.

- They frequently make excuses for their partner's behavior and negative treatment of them.

- They may have a series of injuries, with vague or suspicious excuses.

- They may frequently miss work or school, again with vague or suspicious excuses.

- They may be isolated from friends or family. They may rarely see others besides their partner.

The full range of warning signs of IPV, including signs that you are working with someone who may be violent with their partner, is beyond the scope of this pocket resource. Talk with your supervisor about learning more about this topic.

A SITUATION THAT INVOLVES POSSIBLE CHILD ABUSE

Child abuse is common, and can include physical, sexual, or emotional abuse or neglect. Estimates suggest that in the United States, five children die every day as a result of child abuse.

Learn and follow the local guidelines for responding to the discovery of child abuse. Talk about them with your supervisor before you uncover situations and have to respond.

Every state in the US has laws mandating professionals to report evidence of child abuse that they become aware of. Common mandated reporters include physicians, social workers, psychologists, counselors, teachers, and police. Peer Specialists, self-help group facilitators, and other people who may not be mandated to report child abuse can report it. Talk with your supervisor and local providers about how to handle situations in which you become aware of possible or likely child abuse. Again, clinical providers often have significant training in assessing and responding to child abuse. Get them involved quickly.

There is a wide range of warning signs of child abuse—a discussion of all of the signs is beyond the scope of this pocket resource. Talk with your supervisor to learn more.

A SITUATION THAT INVOLVES POSSIBLE ELDER ABUSE

Abuse of older adults is also surprisingly common and involves physical, sexual, or emotional abuse, as well as neglect or abandonment, or misuse of the older adult's money or property.

Elder abuse can happen in families or in institutions that care for the elderly. Learn and follow the local and regional guidelines for responding to elder abuse. Talk about them with your supervisor before you uncover situations and have to respond.

Similar to child-abuse laws, there are regional laws mandating health-care professionals to report elder abuse. If you think you are working with someone who might be a victim of elder abuse, contact your supervisor or another available clinician as quickly as possible.

Watch for some of the most common warning signs that may identify victims of elder abuse:

- They may seem depressed or confused.

- They are losing weight for no reason.

- They have trouble sleeping.

- They act agitated or violent.

- They have become withdrawn.

- They stop taking part in activities enjoyed in the past.

- They have unexplained bruises, burns, or scars.

- They look messy; they may have unwashed hair or dirty clothes.

- They display signs of trauma (i.e., rocking back and forth).

- They develop bedsores or other preventable conditions.

BIBLIOGRAPHY

Anonymous, A. (2001). Alcholics Anonymous: The Big Book, Fourth Edition. New York, Alcoholics World Services, Inc.

Barlow, J., A. Turner and C. Wright (2000). "A randomized controlled study of the Arthritis Self-Management Programme in the UK." Health Education Research Theory and Practice **15**: 665-680.

Bright, J. I., K. D. Baker and R. Neimeyer (1999). "Professional and paraprofessional group treatments for depression: A comparison of cognitive-behavioral and mutual support interventions." Journal of Consulting and Clinical Psychology **67**: 491-501.

Chien, W. T., D. R. Thompson and I. Norman (2008). "Evaluation of a peer-led mutual support group for Chinese families of peole wth schizophrenia." American Journal of Community Psychology **42**: 122-134.

Copeland, M. E. (2000). Wellness Recovery Action Plan (WRAP). Dumerston , VT, Peach Press.

Griffiths, C., J. Mitlib, A. Azad, J. Ramsay, S. Eldridge, G. Feder, R. Khanam, R. Munni, M. Garrett, A. Turner and J. Barlow (2005). "Randomized controlled trial of a lay-led self-management programme for Bangladeshi patients with chronic disease " British Journal of General Practice **55**: 831-837.

Heller, T., J. A. Roccoforte, K. Hsieh, J. A. Cook and S. A. Pickett (1997). "Benefits of support groups for families of adults with severe mental illness." American Journal of Orthopsychiatry **67**(2): 187-198.

Holt-Lunstad, J., Smith, T.B., Layton, J.B. (2010). "Social relationships and morality risk: A meta-analytic review". PLos Med, **7**(7), e1000316. doi: 10.1371/journal.pmed.1000316.

Houlston, C., P. K. Smith and J. Jessel (2011). "The relationship between use of school-based peer support initiatives ad the social and emotional well-being of bullied and non-bullied students." Children and Society **25**: 293-305.

Houston TK, Cooper LA and F. DE. (2002). "Internet support groups for depression: a 1-year prospective cohort study." American Journal of Psychiatry **159**(12): 2062-2068.

Humphreys K, Wing S, McCarty D, Chappel J, Gallant L, Haberle B, Horvath AT, Kaskutas LA, Kirk T, Kivlahan D, Laudet A, McCrady BS, McLellan AT, Morgenstern J, Townsend M and W. R. (2004). "Self-help organizations for alcohol and drug problems: toward evidence-based practice and policy." Journal of Substance Abuse Treatment **26**: 151-158.

Humphreys, K. and R. H. Moos (2007). "Can encouraging substance abuse patients to participate in self help groups reduce demand for health care? A quasi-experimental study." Alcoholism: Clinical and Experimental Research **25**: 711-716.

Kantor, D. (2012) Reading The Room: Group Dynamics for Coaches and Leaders. San Francisco: John Wiley & Sons, Inc.

Kaplan, K., Salzer, M.S., Solomon, P., Brusilovskiy, Cousounis, P. (2011). Internet peer support for individuals with psychiatric disabilities: A randomized controlled trial. Social Science and Medicine, **72**: 54-62.

Kaskutas, L. (2009). "Alcoholics Anonymous effectiveness: faith meets science." Journal of Addictive Diseases **28**: 145-157.

Kaskutas, L., J. Bond and H. K (2002). "Social networks as mediators of the effect of Alcoholics Anonymous." Addiction **97**(7): 891-900.

Kelly, J. F., R. L. Stout, M. Magill, J. S. Tonigan and M. E. Pagano (2010). "Mechanisms of behavior change in Alcoholics Anonymous: Does AA improve alcohol outcomes by reducing depression symptoms?" Addiction **105**: 626-636.

Kelly, J. F. and J. D. Yeterian (2011). "The role of mutual-help groups in estending the framework of treatment." Alcohol Research and Health **33**: 350-355.

Kennedy, A., D. Reeves, P. Bower, V. Lee, E. Middleton, G. Richardson, C. Garner, C. Gatley and A. Rogers (2007). "The effectiveness and cost effectiveness of a national lay-led self care support programme for patients with long-term conditions: a pragmatic randomised controlled trial." Journal of Epidemiology and Community Health **61**: 254-261.

Kessler, R. C., K. D. Mickelson and Z. Shanyang (1997). "Patterns and correlates of self-help group membership in the United States." Social Policy **27**(3): 27-46.

Koch, K. & Aden, M. (2014). Guidelines for managing self-help groups: A manual for National MS Sociaty self-help group leaders. National MS Society.

Levi, D. (2011). Group Dynamics for Teams. Thousand Oaks, California: Sage Publications, Inc.

Litt, M. D., R. M. Kadden, E. Kabela-Cormier and N. Petry (2009). "Changing network support for drinking: Network support project two-year follow-up." Journal of Consulting and Clinical Psychology 77(2): 229-242.

Mankowski K.H.E., Moos, R.H. and Finney, J.W. (1999). "Do enhanced friendship networks an,d active coping mediate the effect of self-help groups on substance abuse?" Annals of Behavioral Medicine 21(1): 54-60.

Marmar, C. R., M. J. Horowitz, D. S. Weiss, N. R. Wilner and N. B. Kaltreider (1988). "A controlled trial of brief psychotherapy and mutual-help group treatment of conjugal bereavement." American Journal of Psychiatry 145: 203-209.

Moos, B. and R. H. Moos (2006). "Participation in treatment and Alcoholics Anonymous: a 16-year follow-up of initially untreated individuals." Journal of Clinical Psychology 62: 735-750.

Pagano, M. E., W. L. White, J. F. Kelly, R. L. Stout, R. R. Carter and J. S. Tonigan (2013). "The 10-year course of AA participation and long-term outcomes: A follow-up study of outpatient subjects in Project MATCH." Substance Abuse 34(1): 51-59.

Putnam, R. D. (2000). Bowling alone: The collapse and revival of American community. New York, Sion & Schuster Paperbacks.

Riper H, Spek V, Boon B, Conijn B, Kramer J, Martin-Abello K and S. F. (2011). "Effectiveness of E-self-help interventions for curbing adult problem drinking: a meta-analysis." Journal of Medical Internet Research 13(2): e42.

Salzer, M.S. & Kundra, L.B. (2010). "Liability issues associated with referrals to self-help groups." Psychiatric Services, 61(1), 6-8.

Schulz, U., R. Pischke, G. Weidner, J. Daubenmer, M. Elliot-Eller, L. Scherwtz, M. Bulliner and D. Ornish (2008). "Social support group attendance is related to blood pressure, health behaviours, and quality of life in the Multicenter Lifestyle Demonstrtion Project." Psychology Health and Medicine 13(4): 423-437.

Timko, C., A. Debenedetti and R. Billow (1012006). "Intensive referral to 12-step self-help groups and 6-month substace use disorder outcomes." <u>Addiction</u> **101**(5): 678-688.

Timko, C., A. Sutkowi, R. C. Cronkite, K. Makin-Byrd and R. H. Moos (2011). "Intensive referral to 12-step dual-focused mutual-help groups." <u>Drug & Alcohol Dependence</u> **118**: 194-201.

Walitzer, K. S., K. H. Dermen and C. Barrick (2009). "Facilitating involvement in Alcoholics Anonymous during out-patient treatment: A randomized clincial trial." <u>Addiction</u> **104**(3): 391-401.

Look For The Following Upcoming Titles In This Series:

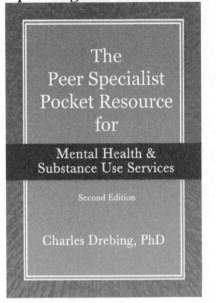

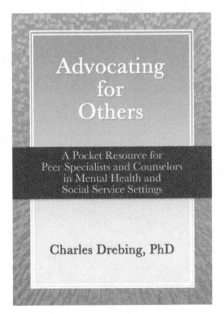

The Peer Specialist Pocket Resource for Mental Health & Substance Use Services, Second Edition

Including Peer Specialists in Health Care Settings is one of the most important developments in the past 30 years. The expanded edition of this pocket resource for Peer Specialists is designed to help you serve effectively as a peer while navigating what is often a complex and confusing clinical setting. Chapters include: Dealing with Critical Situations, Creating and Using Good Recovery Stories, Helping Clients Navigate Healthcare and Social Service Systems.

Advocating for Others: A Pocket Resource for Peer Specialists and Counselors in Mental Health and Social Service Settings

Peer Specialists and counselors are particularly well suited to advocate for change in healthcare and social service organizations on behalf of clients and other stakeholders. This pocket resource is designed to help you develop and deepen your advocacy skills. Chapters include: The Advocate's Stance, Building Support, Common Mistakes, Strategies for Persuasion, Talking the Language of Money, Talking the Language of Quality

.